UNWELL WRITING CENTERS

UNWELL WRITING CENTERS

Searching for Wellness in Neoliberal Educational Institutions and Beyond

GENIE NICOLE GIAIMO

UTAH STATE UNIVERSITY PRESS
Logan

© 2023 by University Press of Colorado

Published by Utah State University Press
An imprint of University Press of Colorado
1624 Market Street, Suite 226
PMB 39883
Denver, Colorado 80202-1559

 The University Press of Colorado is a proud member of
the Association of University Presses.

The University Press of Colorado is a cooperative publishing enterprise supported, in part, by Adams State University, Colorado State University, Fort Lewis College, Metropolitan State University of Denver, University of Alaska Fairbanks, University of Colorado, University of Denver, University of Northern Colorado, University of Wyoming, Utah State University, and Western Colorado University.

∞ This paper meets the requirements of the ANSI/NISO Z39.48-1992 (Permanence of Paper).

ISBN: 978-1-64642-445-0 (hardcover)
ISBN: 978-1-64642-359-0 (paperback)
ISBN: 978-1-64642-360-6 (ebook)
https://doi.org/10.7330/9781646423606

Cataloging-in-Publication data for this title is available online at the Library of Congress.

Cover illustration: Public-domain image from pixabay.com

To my family and to care workers everywhere.

CONTENTS

FOREWORD

Elizabeth H. Boquet
Fairfield University

What a time to be searching for wellness. On the one hand, aren't we all? On the other hand, where would we begin to look?

Do we begin on Sunday evening, when a colleague who is a new chair messages me about requests they have been receiving all weekend that need attention before the next workday? Or on Monday morning, when I pull into the campus parking lot to find a text from a graduate assistant, out sick with a sinus infection, requesting permission to tutor online from home? Maybe when I flip on the lights in the Writing Center and spot the thermometer, still in its packaging, and the fuzzy blanket with the university logo, still folded and tied—a gift from the campus wellness committee (whoever that is), left sometime last year, when we were all working remotely. Does it make sense to start at the end of the day, when the Calm app, to which all university employees were given a free subscription, reminds me to take a minute to breathe? Duly noted.

Genie and I met in the summer of 2019, when we both attended the Dartmouth Summer Institute for Writing Research, a two-week intensive research program. We bonded over our shared appreciation for cozy reading nooks and late-night cups of tea. Neither one of us knew at the time how precious the opportunity to share space for hours and days on end would become, that by the next summer we would be Zooming in rather than settling into professional development spaces. Still, we knew it was a special time, and it was one where I began to learn how deeply invested in writing centers, in research, in wellness, and in social justice Genie was and also what a unique set of skills and experiences she brings to this inquiry.

https://doi.org/10.7330/9781646423606.c000a

In this book Genie charts this interest, deftly managing a mixed-methods approach to her subject, framing the entire project with a compelling autoethnography, tracing her journey through national and local events, through campus partnerships, through the various literatures on workplace wellness and workplace stresses. She reads the writing center as a workplace, training a labor-oriented lens on writing center wellness. Writing centers have been living in an age of austerity (to invoke Nancy Welch and Tony Scott's work) for as long as they have been in existence. Genie positions peer tutor as one of the most precarious labor categories in higher education, as subject as any worker to disaster capitalism's worst effects.

Readers will find in this book a compelling antidote to the "overcoming" narratives that underpin most corporatized wellness efforts. In the early chapters, Genie traces her own journey as a writing center director, building partnerships in response to tutor and student needs, one of which involved work with the campus wellness center. As she begins to recognize the limitations of accepted wellness practices, I heard echoes of Kenneth Bruffee's reflections on the development of Brooklyn College's peer writing tutoring model, which emerged from his observing students' positive responses to peer counseling sessions. Fifty years later, Genie notes the precise opposite reaction among tutors connected to the campus wellness center. Something has come full circle, but what? Genie breaks open the highly individualistic one-to-one model still governing much writing center work and takes a closer look at what's inside.

Like Genie, I can identify in some of my earliest writing center memories a concern with wellness (though I wouldn't have called it that) and perhaps, more to the point, with the well-being of the people in these places. Unlike Genie, I have resisted thinking of writing centers as workplaces. In fact, in many ways, I was drawn to writing centers precisely because they were *not* workplaces—or so I thought. I had been in workplaces, and I didn't like them. Much of my own scholarship underwrites efforts to make writing centers even less like workplaces than they were when I found them. Maybe this was my own response to the increasingly pervasive sense of anxiety tutors and students carried with them to the writing center, my effort to hold space for playfulness, creativity, exploration, and humanity as the space for these qualities was getting increasingly squeezed out of education altogether. And yet, I can't deny that writing centers are indeed workplaces—deeply formative ones. This book challenges me to do more with that information, especially to consider the ways my own resistance to identifying as a manager in the writing center might unintentionally perpetuate some of the toxic effects of a late-stage capitalist workplace. That's a very persuasive argument.

I learned, then, from Genie's early chapters about the history of workplace wellness programs and about the various ways we can identify and address work-related stressors as they present in writing centers. Her own experiences managing both episodic stressors (such as a violent intruder incident on one campus) and chronic stressors (everything from a lack of role clarity to economic insecurity to harassment) in writing centers will be sadly familiar to many readers, but the resources she provides to assist our own inquiries feel concrete and grounding. While those resources include sample wellness surveys, mindfulness exercises, and emergency plans, the most helpful resource is Giaimo's chapter on designing wellness research projects for our own centers. Always we are reminded to situate the inquiry in our own places, to partner with campus populations (tutors especially), and to engage ethically in all research practices.

As I read further, I found Genie giving language and providing evidence for my felt sense of discomfort with wellness rhetoric. More than that, I came to understand the prevailing white logics of corporatized wellness interventions—marketed, as so many of them are, to white women like me. But where was this dawning awareness going to lead? Where, in the end, would it leave me? The final chapter offers some correctives to the apolitical, individualistic presentation of much wellness work, where Genie turns toward Black feminism and Black liberation social movements. In doing so, she invites us to consider metrics of health alongside wellness, disentangling concepts too frequently collapsed.

Since our conversations in the summer of 2019, Genie's exploration of writing centers and wellness has taken unexpected turns, as the best research does, and she has followed the questions where they have led her, which is admirable and ethical. The "searching" in this book's title is genuine, and I appreciate seeing her mind at work, fearlessly, throughout this volume. You will too.

ACKNOWLEDGMENTS

Without peer writing tutors, this project would not have been possible. Peer writing tutors challenged me to think broadly about my administrative work. They also critiqued many of the same neoliberal systems that I critique here in this book. They shared with me their workplace experiences and their visions for creating better and more ethical writing centers. In short, they are the heart of this book in so many ways and I want to acknowledge that fact here. Thank you.

In particular, I want to thank the tutors who jumped on board the wellness research work at Ohio State, which includes Cynthia Lin, Sara Wilder, Carmen Meza, Sam Turner, Michael Shirzadian, Sam Head, Alyssa Chrisman, Dani Orozco, Nicole Pizarro, Chole Heins, Bobby Lowry, and Yanar Hashlamon.

My editor, Rachael Levay: thank you for pushing this project into the world in an incredibly turbulent time. As we both experienced, the wait was long but well worth the product. Thank you for believing in this project from the onset and seeing it through to its completion. It was a pleasure to work with you.

Thank you to Michael Gravina and Katherine O'Brien for reading chapter drafts, discussing concepts from this book, and sharing input on figures and data. You are my rocks. I could not have done this without your love and genuine interest in this work.

And, finally, to my family. My early experiences with work were shaped by you. You have taught me to lead with integrity, to question unethical and unsafe working conditions, and to always believe in myself. There are no words to express what I have learned from you and what I carry with me in my life because of you.

UNWELL WRITING CENTERS

Introduction
WHY WELLNESS?

This book is many years in the making, perhaps my entire career. The exigency for this project likely started long before my first position as an assistant professor and writing center director at a community college on the South Coast of Massachusetts. It started, perhaps, when I volunteered as a preliteracy instructor for women at Rosie's Place in Roxbury, Massachusetts, and worked with unhoused women, predominately from Haiti, trying to pass their citizenship tests. Or perhaps it started when I entered college as a first-generation student and nearly lost my scholarship in my first year because I couldn't seem to figure out how to write academically. Or it may have started long before that, back home in Staten Island, New York, as I watched my single mother go to work sick and injured because she could not afford to stay home and heal. Or it was shaped by 9/11 and the Boston Marathon bombing, which bracketed my educational journey. The lingering trauma of these events profoundly impacted me personally but also impacted how I moved through social and educational spaces. There are many reasons why wellness matters to me—many of which are connected to labor, quality of life, and issues of access and inclusion. There are also reasons why wellness matters to the field of writing center studies, to the broader field of rhetoric and composition, and to higher education.

MY PERSONAL PROFESSIONAL AUTOBIOGRAPHY
I want to open with my personal professional autobiography, which I have carefully meted out until now but which I hope informs the structure and content of this project. It is a bit lengthy, so buckle in. As a newly graduated PhD in 2014, I accepted my first position at Bristol Community College (BCC). There, I was tasked with bringing rigor and high-impact practices back into the Writing Center. The Writing Center had been passed around from temporary administrator to temporary administrator for over a decade. But in its prime, it was a generative

https://doi.org/10.7330/9781646423606.c000b

space for faculty development on writing across the curriculum peda-gogy. As I found out when I arrived, people longed for the days of a powerful and impactful writing center. They regarded the space as faculty-centered and critically important to teaching. Yet, in the decade between the last faculty director and my arrival to campus, something had fundamentally changed. Perhaps because of the precarity of the hiring process, perhaps because of the tension between administra-tion and faculty, perhaps because of the loss of peer tutors, it became a space that was seen as punitive by students and regulatory by faculty. The missing piece, as I saw it, was student engagement. We knew little about who attended the writing center and why. We also lacked student engagement in the writing center beyond the clientele, such as in our staffing model.

My job, as it was communicated to me, was to bring peer tutors back to the writing center. It was also to establish academic and scholarly prac-tices that tethered our writing center to the larger field. Part of this work included revamping the fallow peer-tutoring course. So, in the fall of 2014, 14 students and I embarked on a journey together to "fix" the writ-ing center. For the first few weeks of class, things ran smoothly. Students did the reading. They wrote their reflection logs. They participated with gusto in class. But as we neared the time when students would complete the ethnographic activities that were part of the course's capstone, things fell apart. Students in the training course struggled to schedule appointments. They failed to observe sessions because of the dispropor-tionate level of cancelations and unfilled appointments. Their attempts to engage with the Writing Center failed on multiple levels because of administrative or cultural issues.

So we went back to the drawing board and created a survey about students' perceptions of the Writing Center (Giaimo, 2017). I don't want to go too much into the details because I have written about this before, but this project opened doors that, at the time, I had not really anticipated. Of course, the study had great outcomes for the student researchers (Giaimo, 2019), and we also learned more detailed informa-tion about the culture of writing and the culture of engagement with the Writing Center on campus. From this information, we changed training, marketing, hiring, and even our tutoring practices. We used data in an informed way to positively influence the writing center—which was a goal of mine and, by proxy, of the tutoring course. This was the first large-scale programmatic assessment that I did outside of graduate school, and it taught me how important local institutional context and culture, as well as site-specific need(s), are to doing writing center research.

THE LESS POSITIVE VERSION OF MY
PROFESSIONAL AUTOBIOGRAPHY

This, however, is the positive framing of that experience. At the time, I naively believed that data was the main and perhaps the only way to combat institutional inertia and other issues. Yet all the data in the world could not prepare me for my work as a writing center administrator at BCC. The truth is that underneath the surface of trying to figure out how to make the Writing Center a more hospitable place to students as well as to tutors, there were tensions that I was completely unprepared to handle. There was, of course, the body of faculty who resisted change. There was also the tension of navigating a position that was only partially in the labor union and the attendant issues of stepping into the minefield of grudges between the administrative and faculty communities. There was the struggle to bring professional (adjunct) tutors on board with change and, ultimately, to encourage them to curtail habits harmful to student engagement, such as copyediting. And there was the student population itself—one in which over 70% of students were Pell Grant recipients, worked full time, and were first generation themselves.

Some of these challenges were ones I anticipated—especially around the high need of the student population. I knew these challenges personally as a working-class first-generation student who also qualified for a Pell Grant. But there were more insidious wellness-based issues that lurked among the workaday happenings at the college. In class one day, my students and I were discussing the "What If?" chapter in the *Longman Guide to Peer Tutoring*. When encouraged to discuss their own "what if" scenarios, pertinent to the school, a student raised their hand and asked:

"What if the student is under the influence?"

"Under the influence of what?" I replied.

The student then told us a story about working with someone who was drunk during course-based tutoring. Realizing that *Longman Guide* hadn't prepared us for many of the realities of working with a nonresidential population in one of the poorest and underemployed regions of Massachusetts, I had to rethink my writing center pedagogy. While I had some personal experiences that were like those of my students and could understand some of what they were going through, my training didn't equip me well enough to deal with many of the realities of my community college students' experiences. If anything, I had tried to separate my life experiences and personal identity from my professional one—something I picked up in graduate school likely due to class-based micro- and macroaggressions. This bifurcation hurt, and when I realized that I needed to draw upon my personal well of experiences and resources and stitch myself together in order to support my tutors, I understood how much we give up—emotionally, personally, even cognitively—to do academic work. Wellness (talking about it, examining it, identifying where it does and does not arise), I have come to realize, is one of the missing links in that chain of professionalization, and its absence causes all kinds of issues later on down the line when our well-being, affect, physicality, or material circumstances are threatened while at work.

The ways in which student tutors navigate situations that suddenly shift and become scary or disorienting has reminded me how I had to learn these things on my own—both in my writing center work and my teaching work. As a tutor, I received no training for how to respond to a graduate student who dropped a 300-page dissertation on the table in front of me and demanded that I edit it because her defense was in a week. I received no training to respond to the student who disrupted my class and yelled in my face about not wanting to read poetry. I received no training for the student whose friend committed suicide and who cried as he explained to me why he was struggling so much in class. In these and other situations, as a writing center administrator and educator, I followed my gut. But, for every person who is willing to ask a student to leave class because they are being disruptive, or who comforts a crying student after receiving their permission to hug them, or who confidently rejects demands to copyedit a dissertation, there are many more who struggle to respond, who respond inappropriately, or who respond in ways they are uncomfortable with. This is not the educators' fault; it is our field's failure to train us.

A NEW "NORMAL"?

At BCC, my search for wellness-related research in writing center work started with assessment but also led me to the work of others concerned with well-being in writing center contexts. Degner et al.'s (2015) piece "Opening Closed Doors" was a watershed moment in writing center research on wellness. The article focuses on the mental health concerns that tutors experience and how this impacts their work in writing centers. Following its publication, I started teaching this article in my tutor training courses, and I ran trainings that engaged with this piece as well as center- and college-specific "what if" scenarios. I took to heart the article's call to focus on mental health concerns and other areas of wellness in tutor training and began to expand my own arsenal of wellness resources. Because of my lack of professional training—among other more personal factors I only later identified—I never felt like what I was doing was enough.

In August 2016, when I became the director of the Writing Center at The Ohio State University (OSU), my work evolved. I was now at the third-largest school in the United States, where support services struggled to keep up with demand. Also, the 2016–2017 academic year was especially chaotic and stressful. Throughout the fall, the presidential election—with its heightened and racist rhetoric—profoundly affected many staff and students at the Writing Center. Instances of hate crimes and hate speech rose, both on campus and off. In early November 2016, Donald Trump was elected. A few weeks after that, OSU had a knife attack that was initially described as an active shooter situation that shut down the campus while the Writing Center was operating. In late January 2017, Trump's Muslim ban created confusion for many of our clients and tutors who were attending school on a visa. Still after that, in early February 2017, Reagan Tokes—an Ohio State student—was murdered. Arriving at OSU, I found myself once again unprepared for the complex wellness issues that arose in and around my center, whether that was managing the emotional fallout from Trump's executive orders or responding to the campus lockdown or fielding other tragedies on and around campus. While many of these crises weren't happening directly in the Writing Center, they still affected the students who worked at and attended the center. Once again, as I did at BCC, I turned to research and assessment to learn if these highly stressful events were impacting tutors in the Writing Center.

In the 2019–2020 academic year, I found myself in a new institutional context—an undergraduate liberal arts college—and facing yet another kind of unanticipated crisis. The COVID-19 pandemic has upended how we go about our daily lives. How we work (or are unable to work), how we socialize, how we feel and function. Suddenly, issues of wellness that were only gestured at in faculty meetings and in college emails are now everywhere. We worry for students' mental health, and for good reason, as mental health issues have been skyrocketing (Anderson, 2020). We talk about all kinds of burnout and fatigue. We see how prolonged stress, compounded with chronic illness, can have deleterious effects on our quality of life. Wellness—or lack thereof—is suddenly out there for everyone to see.

Even though I tried to get ahead of every conceivable crisis, despite my best laid plans, I saw myself once again in charge of a new writing center—this time at Middlebury College—during a time of upheaval. After switching jobs several times and reading about the experiences of other writing program administrators who have experienced mass shooting events (Clinnin, 2020) and natural disasters (Schlachte, 2020), as well as marking that this is not the first but second worldwide crisis I've weathered (I started graduate school during the 2008 recession), I realize that this might simply be the new normal of education work—especially writing administration work—where crises create wellness issues that affect our work in unanticipated ways. We must, then, be preventative in our thinking, policies, and research but also realize that we simply cannot anticipate every crisis coming down the pike. We are facing the effects of disaster capitalism, and the fallout from decades of neoliberal policies made at the educational and governmental levels, which are made worse by intersecting crises like climate change, income inequity, systemic racism, and a host of other issues. Like the one-two punch of the pandemic, where the public health crisis was followed by an economic crisis, these issues are complex and multivalanced. Yet if we create assessment-driven and activist-informed heuristics for how to address issues of wellness in our workplaces, we can at least begin to understand our positionality and responses during moments of great upheaval. As Naomi Klein argues in her book, when crises hit, and we are "psychologically unmoored and physically uprooted" (2007, p. 21), the possibility of exploitation is greatest. To push back against such opportunistic neoliberalism is yet another kind of fight for wellness.

THE RHETORIC OF WELLNESS IN NONACADEMIC CONTEXTS

Our field has a wellness problem, perhaps because our society does too. Until recently, conversations about wellness have been rare except in certain fields, such as the helping professions and activist work. Yet, in the last five years, we have seen an explosion of material touting wellness and self-care practices. Most articles are published in popular publications such as the *New York Times*'s "Bringing Wellness to Your Life" set of articles (n.d.), the *Washington Post Live*'s "Be Well" corporate wellness stories (2021), or wellness influencers and accounts on social media platforms like Instagram. While most wellness media focuses on food, exercise, and other lifestyle habits, wellness rhetoric is infused into everything from self-help (how to be a better friend, how to be bored, how to be an intentional eater/drinker) to career advice (how to advocate for a raise, how to leave a toxic work situation), to how to manage one's emotionality (and productivity) during the pandemic. Yet in academia, which many of us acknowledge is a profession that is also "unwell," we are only just getting around to engaging with wellness. For my part, I have read and, in some cases, helped bring forth this scholarship on wellness and care in writing center work (Giaimo & Hashlamon, 2020). Other scholars, such as those in the recently published *The Things We Carry: Strategies for Recognizing and Negotiating Emotional Labor in Writing Program Administration* (Wooten et al., 2020), are also preoccupied with issues of wellness—be they physical, psychological, emotional, material, or otherwise—that arise in writing administration work.

OVERWORKED, UNDERPAID, AND BURNT OUT: "UNWELL" WRITING CENTER WORKERS

As I have continued my research in this area—and counter to much of the commercialized wellness rhetoric that is thrown at us through social media, news outlets, HR and institutional wellness programs, and for-profit educational companies—I have come to see stories about wellness as stories that are also about labor rights, such as how our field professionalizes us or how our educational institutions press upon us to be "everything to everyone." Before entering academia, I did not anticipate all of the helping work I would come to be expected (or pressured) to do. At different points in my career, I have had to do the work of a therapist, a financial advisor, a risk manager and emergency planner, a building coordinator, an advocate, a human resources liaison, a janitor, and a nonprofit volunteer. This is not to say anything of the nonhelper positions I have taken up such as web manager, publicist and marketer, outreach coordinator, graphic designer, editor, event planner, etc. And, looking back, I have taken on these jobs willingly, for the most part. I have crawled under dusty furniture to tighten bolts, I have done wayfinding throughout my campus and developed center signage, and I have edited my websites with gusto. I have comforted grieving students, I have helped students who were suicidal seek resources, I have been a mandatory reporter of sexual assault, and I have supported students through mental and material crises. And, again, I have done so willingly because I was socialized into this work by receiving support from my faculty and staff mentors. I came to see this work as part of the job of educators.

Yet this work—much of it focused on wellness-related issues—takes a toll on one's well-being. Writing center administrators are often heroic and idealistic people, true believers, who go far above and beyond their duties to support students and their staff members. I have heard many stories about new and not-so-new writing center administrators (WCAs) working long hours, weekends, and holidays to make sure their centers are running well. I, myself, have regularly put in 60-plus-hour work weeks, especially in the first year of each new job (which amounts to a lot of additional work considering I am currently directing my fourth writing center!). And my experience isn't novel, as Wooten et al. note in a chapter on overwork and emotional labor (2020, p. 270). In fact, as faculty become more advanced in their career, it seems they work even longer hours. This labor is also not distributed equally across all academics with faculty of color, LGBTQIA+ faculty, and women taking on far more of this burden than their counterparts.

Yet despite this overwork—where our time is taken up by meetings, responding to emails, mission creep, and administrative service—the field of writing center studies is reluctant to label this work "managerial" (Heckelman, 1998) and has struggled to fit such work in academia's frameworks for promotion. Writing center administrators are, however, often managers *par excellence*. Perhaps because we were trained in the trenches, we are good at rolling up our sleeves and getting things done; however, we lack systemic managerial training and, therefore, struggle with emotional labor and other hidden work expectations (Caswell et al., 2016), as well as burnout.

Our field pays little attention, except in abstract ways, to how we are exploited in our work. Perdue et al. (2017) note the precarity of writing center positions in their analysis of job advertisements, which lack standards and often are full of mission- and job-creep duties. Wooten et al. (2020) dedicates an entire edited collection to labor and wellness issues among writing administrators. Currently, however, there are few, if any, articles on tutors' occupational experiences, including wellness-related issues. While scholars have focused on single elements of tutors' wellness experiences, such as guilt (Nicklay, 2012), mental health concerns (Degner et al., 2015), and emotional triggers (Perry, 2016), there are few concrete examples of wellness interventions that holistically support peer tutors' physical, mental, and material well-being. Additionally, and with the exception of the growing scholarship on race and anti-racism, there are few studies that address factors external to the writing center and how these factors impact our tutors. For example, can a writing center be an ethical and wellness-forward place if the larger institution under which it is housed is not? How do we account for and recognize the stress that local and national events can cause in our centers? This book offers an intervention into these matters.

I have frequently turned to the field to respond to questions like the ones I share above and that arise in my writing center. Many times, I have come away empty-handed. There is little research on how peer tutors experience and characterize their work, how emotional labor factors into tutoring work, or how to develop empirical research questions related to tutor experience and development. In many ways, this book is the one that I wished was available as I searched for ways to better prepare my tutors but also to systemically explore what I saw going on underneath the surface of tutoring and writing center work. It is also the book I wish had been handed to me as a new writing center director or even a new graduate tutor.

My career has taught me hard-learned lessons in understanding how writing center directors (WCDs) are overworked, underpaid, understaffed, and constantly responding to micro and macro crises, to say nothing of micro- and macroaggressions that result from our personal identity markers. These experiences leave us stressed out, burnt out, and questioning. They also leave us little room to consider the more marginalized workers around us, like peer tutors. Research is finally catching up with the lived experiences of WCDs. We are questioning our status, our professional identities (Wooten et al., 2020), and whether our jobs are viable ones to stay in long term (Caswell et al., 2016). Little attention, however, is given to tutors' affective, material, physical, and psychosocial experiences, which I see as a complex network of wellness issues that result from neoliberal policies or from precarities that are created by neoliberalist values. This book offers a deep analysis of occupationally specific phenomena that arise in writing center work; from my research, I have found that many of these issues are ones of wellness. While I argue that the writing center is unwell for many reasons, including how our administrative jobs are perceived and constructed, this book examines the experiences, preferences, feelings, and thoughts of some of the most marginalized workers in writing centers today: peer tutors.

CHAPTER BREAKDOWN

The following chapters are organized in a way that reflects my journey as a writing center director and administrator. It begins with an exigency that I was neither prepared to address nor fully cognizant I was addressing until I was well into the thick of things during my first position, which is: how do I as an administrator identify and respond to the many different issues of wellness that arise in my writing center? These issues are not only ones that are centered on wellness; they are issues of wellness *that arise in an occupational setting*. Therefore, these wellness issues are in the literal sense also labor issues.

This book tells the story of my personal journey to secure wellness in my center, especially for my tutors (it is only quite recently that I realized how large and unfair a task I had charged myself with). Throughout these chapters, I share data from a longitudinal assessment conducted in a Land-Grant R1 institution regarding tutors' experiences of wellness training interventions, their attitudes toward the writing center as a workplace, and their abilities to navigate stressful situations—both inside and outside of the writing center. I also share training documents, emergency planning documents, and several wellness-specific interventions developed from anti-racist, labor-centered, and occupational theories. Findings from my assessment made me recognize the critical role labor plays in tutors' workplace feelings, attitudes, and behaviors. Workplace policies that address labor conditions need to be explicitly paired with any wellness work in the center. Otherwise, this work would be a half-hearted attempt at boosting morale without any appreciable investment on the part of the institution. So, in this way, the research study led me to this larger topic of exploitation and how wellness is only one corrective to such issues in the workplace.

The book begins, however, with **Searching for Wellness**. Once I realized that issues of wellness profoundly impact tutors—and their work—I sought occupational interventions in an institutional setting, such as wellness programs that were touted as preventatives for mental health concerns and other psychosocial issues that students regularly confront. From there, I was introduced to positive psychology—the latest in a long line of workplace wellness programs. Chapter 1 traces the history of workplace wellness programs up through the current day and locates the rise in popularity of these programs within a complicated nexus of workforce development and retention needs, as well as austerity-minded business-logic that promotes toxic bootstrap rhetoric and individualistic change as cost-saving measures. Programs in higher education are not immune to this trend, with several colleges and universities adopting one such program that relies on positive psychology to provide students with wellness support. I share assessment findings from tutors on their experiences of a positive psychology-focused workplace wellness program. Chapter 2 examines factors that lead to occupational stress more broadly, as well as government and international standards for mitigating occupational stress. I then turn to writing center research to understand how our field talks about and conceptualizes stress. Finally, I share study findings on how tutors at my writing center experience work-related stress (internal to the writing center) and external stress of different kinds such as longer-term political stress, and punctuated stress related to emergencies or crises. Chapter 3 and the final part of the first section provides a deeper dive into the methodology underpinning my longitudinal research on tutor wellness and provides guidance on how to conduct such empirical research on wellness at other institutions.

The second section of the book, **Finding Wellness**, provides concrete examples of how to support wellness in the writing center through mindfulness and wellness interventions that tutors favorably rated in my research study (Chapter 4). However, alongside training interventions, I also include policy interventions that are centered on fair labor practices and that I hope administrators will consider implementing as they develop their own wellness interventions. In Chapter 5, I trace the history of emergency planning and risk assessment—especially in higher education—to contextualize and ground the development of an emergency and risk management plan in my writing center, which, I argue, is critical for finding wellness in one's own center. Drawing from my experience of an active shooter alert, as well as several other crises, I provide resources and guidance on creating this critical document and attendant policies around post-crisis response and reflection.

The final two chapters and the conclusion of this book comprise Part III, Looking to the Future of Wellness. Chapter 6 provides an overview of the history of research on emotional labor before turning to research on this topic in writing center studies, which I pair with training resources for identifying and discussing emotional labor in individual centers. I then define burnout—which results, in part, from unchecked emotional stressors in the workplace—and argue that our field's strained relationship with the managerial aspects of our work, paired with austerity measures in the neoliberal university, can produce profound worker burnout. I end with a call to action for the field to develop more ethical models of writing center administration that consider how class and race affects our relationship to our work and our engagement with and responses to emotional labor. In Chapter 7, I trace the history of wellness work that connects wellness to the Civil Rights Movement and its focus on community-based and wraparound healthcare as critical to dismantling racism and creating empowerment and autonomy in Black communities. I then discuss the extension of this work into Black feminism through figurations of radical care and self-care work. In decolonializing the origins of wellness work and situating it in communal, radical, and pro-Black social movements, I aim to demonstrate how critically situating wellness work also contributes to anti-racist wellness models. To that end, I share resources and action items for supporting underrepresented staff in writing centers while also challenging exclusionary and ahistorical wellness programs that center whiteness and comfort over safety for BIPOC staff members.

I conclude the book with how we might envision the future of writing center work as one informed by wellness and care interventions. Along the way, I include data from previous research projects, as well as previously unpublished findings. Each chapter begins with an autobiographical narrative that frames my thinking on wellness work in writing centers, which has been shaped by my lived experiences as a writing center director or associate director at four very different institutional types (R1 private, two-year college, R1 public, and selective liberal arts college). While I locate my research on workplaces and wellness in writing centers, this research can just as easily be carried out in other workplaces inside and outside of higher education. And findings and best practices that emerge from this work can be easily applied in teacher-mentor situations, in laboratories, among sports teams, and in first-year orientation and writing programs. In short, in whatever blurry spaces that students occupy as both students and workers, and in those spaces where issues of wellness leave deep marks on individuals as well as the collective, this book's findings are applicable.

WELLNESS RESEARCH IN WRITING CENTER STUDIES

Although there is not currently a lot of published research on wellness, care, and labor in writing center work, that does not mean that larger conversations about these topics are not taking place in our field. To the contrary, the 2018 East Central Writing Centers Association Conference, held at Ohio State, saw roughly 100 presentations and nearly 300 attendees present on wellness, care, and labor ethics in writing center work. Also, in 2018, the South Central Writing Centers Association hosted a conference on mindfulness at the writing center. Recently, *WLN: A Journal of Writing Center Scholarship* published a special issue on wellness and care in writing center work. And, in the first digital edited collection published by *WLN*, Featherstone et al. (2019) published a chapter on a mindfulness training intervention, along with assessment data on its efficacy. Finally, another digital edited collection, of which I am the editor, on wellness and care work in writing centers was published in early 2021. And, in the broader field of composition studies, research on mindfulness (Mathieu, 2016), contemplative writing practices (Wenger, 2015), and emotional labor (Sano-Franchini, 2016) all indicate a sustained interest in applying wellness theories and practices to writing administration and pedagogical practices. Additionally, several projects are in the pipeline, so to speak, on emotional labor, such as Concannon and Morris's edited collection on affect (Parlor Press, forthcoming).

Wooton et al.'s book on emotional labor in writing program administration was published in fall 2020 and became the subject of several book clubs and the plenary for the International Writing Centers Association 2021 Collaborative. And *The Working Lives of New Writing Center Directors* (Caswell et al., 2016) has critically informed research on emotional labor, up to this point, in writing center studies. So, this book is in good company, alongside the interests and scholarship of hundreds of writing center practitioners and compositionists. We, as a field, are hungry to be well—to have wellness centered and upheld in our work—however, the socioeconomic contexts underpinning the sudden explosion of interest in wellness has been left sadly under-examined, as have the historical and political origins of wellness sub-fields like mindfulness, self- and community-care, and workplace safety. We need an institutional history of wellness that situates it in progressive political movements that demanded safety, fair wages, and care for communities of color and the working class.

Broadly speaking, more discussions about the labor that we perform in our field need to be had at all levels—regional, national, international, and, of course, local. And, while some administrators may still believe that writing can somehow be divorced from the emotions and experiences of clients, many more recognize that tutors (and educators more broadly) have been performing wellness work with and for their clients for as long as writing centers have been around. Even the formalization of writing centers, in the current moment, was galvanized in an emotionally heightened period in our educational system: during the open access movement. Writing centers became part of a systemic support model offered in higher education institutions around the country at a time in which institutions, administrators, and educators argued that newcomers to higher education needed additional academic support (Boquet, 1999). Framing writing center work within a deficit education model—one that we still carry forward when we use the language of "help" to describe the work that writing centers perform—elides the historical roots of our labor as emotionally charged, stressful, and rooted in a white racial habitus. As Asao Inoue (2015) describes it, a racial habitus is "a set of structuring structures, some marked on the body, some in language practices, some in the ways we interact or work, write, and read, some in the way we behave or dress, some in the processes and differential opportunities we have" (p. 43). The pedagogical and occupational origins of writing centers are steeped in a white racial habitus and have helped to frame how we justify our work structures as much as we do our workplace practices.

It should come as no surprise, then, that tutors characterize and describe the work that they do in far more complex ways than scholars often do (Giaimo et al., 2018). Tutors use emotionally charged language in their session notes and express feelings of doubt, misgiving, and even shame when describing their labor in these notes. Through conducting a corpus analysis of a year's worth of session notes, I was able to trace the invisible labor that tutors perform and to locate it within affective work centered on the language of failure. In using wellness as a heuristic through which to frame writing center labor, we can consider different administrative maneuvers we may take to mitigate tutors' complicated or downright negative experiences in their work. Of course, training interventions and policies are only developed after we acknowledge and study what is going on at our centers. To me, research is a useful way in which to ground wellness interventions in evidence-based practices, but it is not the only way to do this work. We also need to draw upon pro-labor and anti-racist policies and practices to do this work.

Other scholars have approached studying writing center phenomena from a similarly research-based inquiry. As Mark Hall (2017) notes in his excellent book, *Around the Texts of Writing Center Work*, "Examination of everyday documents . . . illuminates the theories that underpin and motivate writing centers" (p. 4). It is the quotidian nature of writing center work that Hall attempts to make visible and render scholarly. Through analyzing different documents, he can theorize writing center work. Yet the work itself is not necessarily only theoretical or scholarly, nor is it only informed by scholarship; it is embodied and affective (Lawson, 2015); it is material; it is emotional.

WELLNESS IS NOT A CURE-ALL FOR THE NEOLIBERAL UNIVERSITY

The work we do, however, is also political and intimately tied to our identities and relative positionality within the broader institution. We need to recognize both the liminality of peer tutors—their liminality as students and staff—and we need to set up robust responses to caring for their wellbeing while also recognizing how easily wellness interventions can be coopted by the neoliberal academy (Monty, 2019). In my search for wellness for my tutors—and for myself—I came across several corporate and institutional interventions that placed expectations for success and wellness primarily on the individual. In addition to culling from institutional histories of workplace wellness programs, I referred to national and international guidelines for workplace standards for safety and wellness. Yet even as I drew from power structures such as higher education, government agencies, or international organizations, I realized that neoliberalism—a political approach that favors free-market capitalism, deregulation, and reduction in government spending—underpins much of the creation of these policies and structures. My research—and my tutors' responses to our developing wellness project—taught me that there are very few quick fixes to wellness issues in workplaces because these issues are systemic and because they are informed by internal and external factors that are not entirely in our control.

In higher education, I believe, we are always fighting against the alluring fantasy of neoliberal wellness, which is that if the individual puts enough policies in place; if they spend just a little more personal time; if they trace out and anticipate enough eventualities; if they, in other words, do more and more and more with less and less and less, then our educational spaces (and our students and tutors) will be remade and be well. For the past 40 years, the United States has been dominated by such neoliberal thinking, which has led to policies and practices that many believe improve "national conditions for free markets, increasing global competition, and establishing new national and global economic configurations" (Vazquez & Levin, 2018). Yet these policies have resulted in "drastic cuts to state supported social services and programs, the extension [of] an economic rationality to cultural, social, and political spheres, and the redefinition of the individual from a citizen to an autonomous economic actor" (Saunders, 2010, p. 42). As neoliberalism became the dominant ideology in US politics and business, it also infiltrated higher education through management policies informed by "new public management," which touts smaller, leaner management that is customer-focused (Olssen & Peters, 2005), and that drastically revised the "core professional academic values" of the institution and its faculty (Vazquez & Levin, 2018). As Vazquez and Levin (2018) note,

> The infiltration of neoliberal ideology into public research universities, particularly the increase of managerialism, surveillance, and accountability, is enabled by the assumption that there is no alternative to symbolic violence, precariousness in work conditions, or denial of humanity for academic professionals. The consequences of the rise of symbolic violence affects the psycho-emotional life and well-being of faculty members, causing stress, anxiety, feelings of powerlessness, loss of autonomy, and uncertainty in relation to their profession (Vazquez & Levin, 2010).

Here, Vazquez and Levin (2018) identify the ways in which neoliberal ideology has harmed academia and the professorate. The economic and political aims of this ideology have, of course, come home to roost in our educational institutions. We see this in mobile foodbanks on our campuses. We see this in the rates of suicide and mental health concerns among our students. We see this in the increased number of mass shooting events on campuses around the country. We see this in the rise of adjunct labor and the disappearance of tenure track lines. We see this in the closure of entire departments—or schools—and the furloughs, retrenchments, and layoffs that accompany these economic decisions.

In writing centers, we are continuously faced with the results of neoliberal ideology and policy. In many ways, it drives our customer-service model of support and how we assess our success. It is possible, with the boom in wellness research on subjects like emotional labor, burnout, triggers, etc., that we as a field are sick of being unwell. As austerity measures at the university level increase—especially with the economic fallout from the pandemic—we are all feeling the squeeze more profoundly in the current era. Our turn to wellness, then, might be a localized response to austerity. What better response to the dehumanizing mechanistic and profit-driven ideologies of neoliberalism than the humanizing, values-driven ideology of wellness? While a good response; it should not be the only response. We need to hold our institutions accountable and resist plugging all gaps that neoliberalism creates with further exploitation of ourselves and others.

So, even though this book argues for several wellness interventions in the writing center, it asks practitioners to think carefully before they develop and implement wellness programs in their educational spaces. It asks practitioners to consider the interconnectedness of workplace wellness interventions and advocacy work. It asks practitioners to assess their wellness work and to listen to their tutors as they redesign their interventions. In short, this book guides practitioners through some hard-learned lessons about neoliberal wellness programs and how to develop sustainable and more ethical models that consider not only wellness programs but also workplace policies. I hope this book will help administrators and tutors alike to smartly intervene and to better support the wellness of their centers and their own wellness, but also, in the immortal words of Kenny Rogers (1978), "Know when to hold 'em, know when to fold 'em, know when to walk away, and know when to run."

PART I

Searching for Wellness

1

WRITING CENTERS AND THE HISTORY OF WORKPLACE WELLNESS PROGRAMS

OPENING NARRATIVE

I began developing my own workplace wellness programs long before I knew what a workplace wellness program was; first at BCC and then as the new writing center director at The Ohio State University. My wellness training interventions (Appendix A) were developed out of what was at the time rather limited scholarship on wellness. In the first workshop at OSU, I introduced tutors to "Opening Closed Doors" (Degner et al., 2015). Excited and a little nervous, I arrived on campus in mid-August ready to have an open and earnest discussion about mental health concerns with my new staff. Yet as I stood at the head of a room of 45 silent undergraduate and graduate tutors, I realized how important community building is to discussing topics of wellness.

When they did finally start talking (and it was a good 10 minutes before they did), the tutors resisted discussing mental health within the context of tutor experience. Rather, they focused on students' experiences of mental health concerns and ways they could be of support. At the time, I thought the tutors' reticence came from their unfamiliarity with each other and with me. What I came to learn over time, however, is that many tutors struggled with mental health concerns and were, at the same time, worried that disclosure would cost them their job. This is yet another neoliberal value that one can trace into writing centers where the onus for performance is placed squarely on the individual with little thought to their well-being and personal experiences and how these things affect their work. So, instead of talking about tutors, we brainstormed the different needs that clients may bring into the writing center and then we worked on responses to those specific scenarios. After discussion, we developed a list of resources available at OSU for students, which included on-campus and off-campus counseling, legal services, suicide prevention training, active shooter training, and so on. In large schools, particularly ones as

https://doi.org/10.7330/9781646423606.c001

sprawling as Ohio State, it is critical to have a robust and up-to-date list of resources that tutors can use to make referrals. Upon opening the writing center, I noticed there were out-of-date fliers for counseling services, disability services, and OSU student resources; I wondered how many tutors had given these documents to clients in good faith only for the clients to be sent to the wrong building or to call a disconnected phone line. One of the first projects I had a tutor perform during the downtime of the early semester was requesting current informational materials from these offices. We also shared these materials at all our sites, including an updated university-wide handout, "Guide to Assist Distressed Individuals" (The Ohio State University, n.d.).

I mention this early wellness-resource "housekeeping" activity for a couple of reasons. First, before engaging in a discussion about mental health concerns among tutors, it makes sense to scope out the current support networks in place on campus. Second, connecting with student support services is an easy way to help tutors prepare for cross-referral. However, as I came to learn over time, just because a university *seems* to have student resources does not mean that these resources are accessible or robust. The wait time for counseling, for example, ranged from 3 to 11 weeks during the time that I worked at OSU. Many students expressed their frustration with what they felt was an inadequate institutional response to their needs. Later on, they also expressed distrust of institutionalized care programs.

In the early days of my new position, however, I had no such context for workplace wellness programs or which ones were successful. So, instead of developing more workshops on my own, I turned to the wellness center on campus. After a series of discussions, we arranged for wellness ambassadors to attend tutors' weekly mentorship groups for a multiweek series of discussions on the nine dimensions of wellness (Table 1.1), implicit and explicit motivation, and personal development (The Ohio State University, 2017). Here, I thought, tutors could open up about their own experiences with wellness and move toward more personal discussions. I also participated in these conversations, as I ran one of the mentorship groups.

Tutors engaged in three one-hour-long wellness sessions in coordination with the Wellness Center. Training included discussing different elements of wellness and results from the psychometric personality test VIA Character Strengths Survey, which was developed in part by the psychologist Martin Seligman (VIA Institute on Character, n.d.). The second meeting covered goal-setting and extrinsic and intrinsic motivation, by engaging in different writing activities in which members shared their

Table 1.1. Nine dimensions of wellness and attendant definitions

Dimension	Definition
Emotional Wellness	The emotionally well person can identify, express, and manage the entire range of feelings and would consider seeking assistance to address areas of concern.
Career Wellness	The professionally well person engages in work to gain personal satisfaction and enrichment, consistent with values, goals, and lifestyle.
Social Wellness	The socially well person has a network of support based on interdependence, mutual trust, and respect and has developed a sensitivity and awareness toward the feelings of others.
Spiritual Wellness	The spiritually well person seeks harmony and balance by openly exploring the depth of human purpose, meaning, and connection through dialogue and self-reflection.
Physical Wellness	The physically well person gets an adequate amount of sleep, eats a balanced and nutritious diet, engages in exercise for 150 minutes per week, attends regular medical check-ups and practices safe and healthy sexual relations.
Financial Wellness	The financially well person is fully aware of their financial state and budgets, saves, and manages finances in order to achieve realistic goals.
Intellectual Wellness	The intellectually well person values lifelong learning and seeks to foster critical thinking, develop moral reasoning, expand worldviews, and engage in education for the pursuit of knowledge.
Creative Wellness	The creatively well person values and actively participates in a diverse range of arts and cultural experiences as a means to understand and appreciate the surrounding world.
Environmental Wellness	The environmentally well person recognizes the responsibility to preserve, protect, and improve the environment and appreciates the interconnectedness of nature and the individual.

aspirational goals within a SMART (specific, measurable, achievable, relevant, and time-bound) goals framework, and how those goals fit into one or more of the wellness dimensions. The final meeting introduced the concept of "change talk"—an articulation of the reason, desire, and motivation to change a behavior or habit—as well as the transtheoretical model of change (Prochaska & DiClemente, 1982, p. 277; Prochaska et al., 1993, p. 1103), a biopsychosocial model that conceptualizes the process of intentional behavioral change. To articulate change-talk and motivation-to-change, the group engaged in "motivational interviewing," which offers an individual support in their change-talk and in meeting their goals (Miller & Rollnick, 2004, p. 299). During motivational interviewing, we conducted active listening activities that, interestingly, mimicked the agenda-setting stage of consultations.

Looking back on my notes from this wellness program, I notice how much of the framing of wellness coaching focused on the individual and their responsibility to make intentional changes to their habits and behaviors. At the time, I was grateful for any support, so I gave this little thought outside of my brainstorming and reflection notes. Initially, the nine dimensions of wellness appealed to me and seemed to appeal to a few of the tutors in the group. Many expressed desires to set goals that fostered their spiritual, physical, social, and environmental wellness. Tutors talked about connecting more with their spiritual lives, getting more sleep, connecting more with family and friends, and going out into nature more often. From these discussions, I learned a lot about my tutors as holistic people both inside and outside of their writing center work. I was also given a chance, as a new director, to share my own goals and experiences. Most of mine centered around career wellness, intellectual wellness, and physical wellness. Interestingly, the dimensions that appealed to tutors and administrators had little overlap beyond physical wellness, which might be a testament to the different needs that student and administrative workers face.

After the initial round of workplace wellness training, tutors reported dissatisfaction with the program's approach. Some tutors noted that it was too generic to be applicable in workplace settings. Others did not believe that the goals of the program were ethical. Still others felt discomfort sharing their personal experiences, thoughts, and motivations in the workplace. I decided to do an assessment of the tutors and the center, in which I surveyed tutors on their experiences with the institutional wellness program as compared to our in-house trainings and workshops on wellness topics. While the scope of the assessment started out small, I later added questions about tutors' experiences of workplace, institutional, and national stress (and crisis events), as well as questions about tutors' engagement with their work. This project developed organically over the fall 2016 semester, and it started with a few dissatisfied tutors who were brave enough to talk with me openly, as well as my sinking feeling that institutional wellness programs—and positive psychology in particular—weren't effective ways to support the well-being of tutors.

In the past, when I have presented on the dimensions of wellness and our first wellness training intervention at OSU, writing center directors inevitably become excited. They would come up to me after the presentation and ask for more detail and training materials. Over time, however, I have become more reluctant to share this information, as I believe there are serious limitations and biases implicit in the theoretical framework that informs the dimensions of wellness and the attendant trainings that are provided by sanctioned university sources. However, there has always been a connection between psychology and writing center studies, which I think carries over into the current engagement with models such as the dimensions of wellness and other positive psychology interventions in mental health support for students. Additionally, because many administrators are strapped for time and resources, a ready-made wellness model is incredibly appealing, as I can attest to from my own experience in trying to develop wellness trainings in the first few weeks of my job at OSU.

LITERATURE REVIEW
Psychology and Writing Center.Work

The adaptation of positive psychology and personality psychology to writing center wellness training is not the first time that concepts from psychology have been applied to writing center work. Despite its analogical shortcomings, psychology is a lens through which we understand writing center work, perhaps because we define what we do in terms of help and care. The current iteration of many writing center tutorials and the emphasis on nondirective tutoring methods has roots in Rogerian nondirective counseling, a version of psychotherapy (Boquet, 1999, p. 470); the tutoring process has also been compared to psychoanalysis (Murphy, 1989, p. 13). Other scholars have relied on more ambiguous clinical and medical analogies to describe writing tutoring, although these often also have an affective or psychological valence (Morrow, 1991). More recently, writing center studies have focused on transfer of writing knowledge, metacognition, and efficacy (Driscoll & Wells, 2012), which are topics often also found in fields such as educational psychology and scholarship of teaching and learning. More broadly, the field of composition and rhetoric has also relied on the psychology of learning and development "to shore up its claims about language development and acquisition" (Driscoll & Wells, 2012, pp. 469–470).

The Rogerian approach to tutoring—a keystone in early writing center tutoring practice—much like the positive-psychology approach to wellness, places too much expectation for action and change on the individual. As Boquet (1999) notes, Rogerian nondirective tutoring is modeled on "a method which has psychotherapists ask questions in order to draw out their patients, leading to knowledge these clients presumably already possess" (p. 469). This approach is "yet another means for individual students to be held accountable for their own successes as well as for their shortcomings by making students responsible for accessing information which continually eludes them" (p. 470). Whether that information regards writing process, writing strategies, editorial decision-making, or self-motivation in goal-setting, change talk, and personality development, the underlying philosophical framework is similar. And while the Rogerian-inspired tutoring method was criticized as a version of "amateur psychology" (Carino, 1995, p. 107), it still pervades the rhetoric of writing center work (i.e., nondirective, talk-focused, individual-centered, help-centered) and therefore has left its fingerprints all over our field. In some ways, the positive psychology movement's focus on the individual as change agent shares a parallel philosophy. Because of the allure of applying psychological principles to writing center work, this chapter focuses on the development of the positive psychology movement and attempts to unpack some of its more complicated and fraught approaches to development of the self. I hope we do not leap into utilizing institutional wellness approaches even though a growing number of colleges and universities have already switched to them for their own wellness initiatives on campus.

POSITIVE PSYCHOLOGY AND UNIVERSITY STUDENT WELLNESS INITIATIVES

The OSU student-wellness training takes as its foundation the nine dimensions of wellness developed by the positive psychology (PP) movement, which was popularized by psychologist Martin Seligman around 2000, when, as president of the American Psychological Association, he chose it as a focus area for the organization (n.d.). Seligman is the director of the Positive Psychology Center at University of Pennsylvania. Positive psychology argues for treating an individual's well-being in a holistic, multidimensional way. For too long, Seligman argues, psychology has been preoccupied with mental illness. Drawing on early research from Maslow that used the term, this field focuses less on human suffering and more on how individuals can live meaningful and fulfilling lives. Martin Seligman and Mihály Csikszentmihályi (2014) published a paper calling to redirect the field of psychology's attention away from pathology and "repairing the worst things in life" and toward "building positive qualities" of an individual:

> The field of positive psychology at the subjective level is about valued subjective experiences: well-being, contentment, and satisfaction (in the past); hope and optimism (for the future); and flow and happiness (in the present). At the individual level, it is about positive individual traits:

the capacity for love and vocation, courage, interpersonal skill, aesthetic sensibility, perseverance, forgiveness, originality, future mindedness, spirituality, high talent, and wisdom. At the group level, it is about the civic virtues and the institutions that move individuals toward better citizenship: responsibility, nurturance, altruism, civility, moderation, tolerance, and work ethic. (p. 5)

Bound up in current rhetoric of "grit" and the culture of positive thinking, positive psychology shares a lineage with other psychological movements of the 19th and 20th centuries, such as mental hygiene, moral psychology, and "New Thought" (Becker & Marecek, 2008, p. 592). While a lot of the research seems to bear a similar resemblance to self-help rhetoric, positive psychology does focus on the different values, virtues, and characteristics that so-called flourishing individuals possess and how to effect similar self-directed positive change in people who do not possess such characteristics.

Becker and Marecek identify a number of issues with the PP movement—namely, its lack of cultural interrogation or exploration of systemic imbalances of power that might be related to its "visions of the good life or with who can or cannot attain it [and] . . . that some segments of the population may 'flourish' at the expense of others" (p. 596). While there are clear philosophical issues with the positive psychology movement—including its focus on a reactive rather than preventive approach to mental well-being and support, as well as its generally uncritical engagement with systemic inequity and the precarity caused by late-stage capitalism—it has become a popular model for institutional wellness support. The nine dimensions of wellness were developed out of the PP movement; they are a cornerstone of OSU's student wellness program. Many other universities across the country (University of North Carolina, Oberlin College, Clark College, UC David, etc.) have also included the dimensions of wellness model in student wellness resources and training.

The student wellness program at OSU is part of a growing suite of support services that colleges and universities offer to students. Some of these services, such as counseling and health centers, have been offered to students for decades, but others, such as the wellness program at OSU, or mindfulness initiatives to support stress reduction, are relatively new. Many of these programs "are designed to improve students' physical and mental health, promote psychosocial and stress management techniques, decrease depression and anxiety, and develop positive health behaviors to enhance students' quality of life" (Franzidis & Zinder, 2019). Yet as Cole et al. (2018) note, meta-analysis of studies on specific interventions that aim to affect student health and wellness, such as alcohol consumption reduction, find little difference in short-term behavior between students who undergo training and the control group and, strikingly, "statistically significantly more alcohol-related problems than controls" in the long-term (p. 686). Because of such findings, Franzidis & Zinder (2019) suggest that "despite the many campus-based wellness programs and services offered, many U.S. students lack the strategies, skills, or support systems to manage stress or change pre-existing behaviors resulting in unhealthy behaviors and poor overall wellness" (p. 57). They advocate for more robust programming and returning to the dimensions of wellness featured in positive psychology to advocate for more targeted and population-specific interventions.

HISTORY OF WORKPLACE WELLNESS PROGRAMS

Student wellness programs share several similarities with workplace wellness programs. Both are part of a multi-billion-dollar occupational wellness industry; both struggle to empirically prove their success; both are relatively new trends in occupational spaces; and both are rooted in a paternalistic philosophy that seeks to optimize labor through industrial means. While wellness programs often characterize their intentions through uplift rhetoric that supports so-called thriving individuals, these programs were largely established to save corporations money through decreasing employee turnover and healthcare costs and increasing productivity.

Employee-focused workplace wellness programs in America span back to at least the 1980s (Call et al., 2009). Early iterations of workplace wellness programs focused on physical, rather than mental, health, providing employee perks such as workplace fitness centers. During the past decade or so, however, more extensive and holistic workplace wellness programs have propagated in part because of provisions in the Affordable Care Act, which provided grants and other support for establishing such programs (Liu et al., 2013; Song & Baicker, 2019). American workplaces are comprised of an increasingly aging and unhealthy workforce, which contributes to rising healthcare costs that do not keep pace with inflation (Beck et al., 2016). Workplace wellness programs, then, are being instituted by employers as a cost-saving corrective to the failing health and associated rising costs of their workforce. Approximately half of employers in the United States offer some kind of workplace wellness program including nutrition support, exercise classes, health information, health screening, health education, chronic disease management, lifestyle behavior modification (such as stress reduction), and employee assistance programs (Dailey et al., 2018, p. 613). Abraham (2019) notes that four out of five large employers offer workplace wellness programs as part of their employee compensation packages and many colleges and universities provide this support as well.

While workplace wellness programs were established in large part to stem the rising costs of providing healthcare to aging and chronically ill workers, there are other attendant reasons for instituting such programs, such as increasing employee retention and productivity (Song & Baicker, 2019) as well as employee morale and performance (Beck et al., 2016). However, research on the efficacy of such programs is incomplete, because of study design issues (Song & Baicker, 2019), and often empirical studies and meta-analyses find little to no change in employee outcomes due to engagement with workplace wellness programs (Liu et al., 2013; Jarman et al., 2015; Abraham, 2019). For example, Nyman et al. (2010) found that while healthcare costs did decrease among employees who participated in disease management, there was no significant change in absenteeism or lifestyle management. Liu et al. (2013) found that their study "did not demonstrate a significant impact of PepsiCo's wellness program on medical care utilization and costs" although their program did not offer disease management support; therefore, they posit that disease management, rather than wellness support, significantly affects participant outcomes (p. 153).

Scholars still know relatively little about the attitudes and perceptions of people who engage in workplace wellness initiatives. There is, however, a lot of research on the demographics and identities of people who are more likely to participate in such programs. Beck et al. (2016) found that participants in the University of Michigan's program were more likely to be "female, white, and in non-union staff positions, as well as those who seek preventive care" (p. 9). Jenkins et al. (2019) had similar findings in their university-based assessment of engagement with workplace wellness programs; they found that participants were largely female, in non-union positions, and earned less than $100,000 a year (p. 882). Both Beck et al. (2016) and Jenkins et al. (2019) note that men and people of color are less likely to participate in employee wellness initiatives, which effectively leaves out large proportions of employees (white men), as well as marginalized employees (people of color). Workplace wellness programs, then, are not universally engaged with and can actually contribute to further alienation of specific employee populations within a workplace.

CRITIQUE OF INSTITUTIONAL WELLNESS PROGRAMS

The capitalistic origins of workplace wellness programs, which aim to optimize labor while also placing the burden of wellness requirements squarely on the individual, as well as the inconclusive evidence surrounding the efficacy of workplace wellness programs, including long-term mitigation of wellness-related issues, are some of the reasons for my eventual decision to forego engagement with institutional wellness programs. As I alluded to earlier, however, the more immediate reason for my movement away from this kind of support was that a number of tutors did not respond favorably to wellness training in that first semester.

WELLNESS PROGRAM ASSESSMENT FINDINGS

Because, as Dailey et al. (2018) note, "we know relatively little about workers' perspectives concerning workplace wellness" (p. 613), I developed and implemented a longitudinal survey with qualitative (open-ended and text-based) and quantitative (Likert scale) questions that tracked tutors' attitudes and engagement with the wellness interventions. Over three years, roughly 45% of the tutor population ($n = 64$) responded to the survey. And, similar to Dailey et al. (2018), I found that employees defined well-being differently than management (p. 614), with tutors wanting opportunities to engage in community-oriented wellness work, as well as writing-center-situated wellness work, as opposed to university wellness programs. Because of this early disconnect between worker and institutional understandings of wellness and the support it requires, initial survey responses to the wellness program were far more negative than in any subsequent survey year (Figure 1.1).

Some tutors noted that the experience of engaging in highly structured and, to them, artificial conversations around wellness was coercive. Others were uncomfortable sharing their experiences in front of me because I was their boss. Still others did not feel like the discussions about wellness extended to any meaningful change in their experiences as writing center tutors. As one tutor wrote, "We aren't counselors, so we should know what to do when people want help, but we shouldn't try to force that intimacy." Tutors also asked for more interaction and to "customize wellness training based on the real and reported problems that consultants have identified, rather than the University's pro-forma presentations designed to limit their legal liability." Some tutors felt that there was a disconnect between writing center work and the institutional wellness program, which focused heavily on goal-setting and its relationship to the

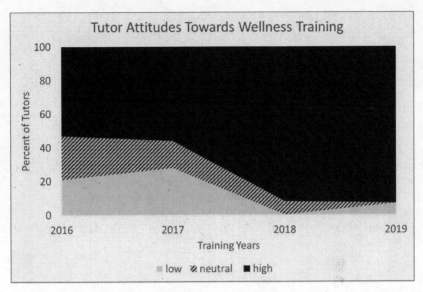

Figure 1.1. Tutors' responses to wellness training by year with low and neutral responses significantly higher in 2016 and 2017 than in 2018 and 2019.

topics of mental health and wellness. Tutors also felt that mental health was not genuinely discussed or addressed during workshop discussions.

In addition to the qualitative responses to the school's wellness training, tutors responded least favorably to the wellness trainings in 2016 and 2017, with a larger percentage of respondents reporting low or neutral attitudes toward wellness training than respondents in 2018 and 2019, where responses were largely favorable (Figure 1.1). In 2016 and 2017, attitudes toward wellness training (Appendix B) show both a wider range of response as well as a more negative agreement response than in 2018 and 2019. These findings are in line with tutors' qualitative responses to the open-ended questions in the survey. They suggest, first, that the early institutional and workplace wellness programs, such as the one I inadvertently established when I partnered the university wellness program, were not well liked by tutors for a variety of reasons. If tutors are suspicious or otherwise disengaged from institutional training, they are unlikely to favorably respond to it. However, wellness training was changed from a workplace model to a more community-centered model, post-2017, which contributed to the positive attitudes toward wellness training tutors reported post-2017 (Figure 1.1).

In addition to negative engagement with the early iterations of our wellness program, we also learned a lot about how likely tutors are to incorporate their wellness training into their everyday tutoring practice.

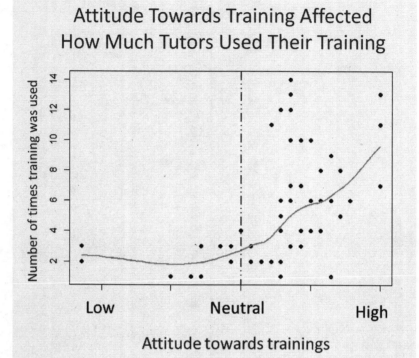

Figure 1.2. Tutors' attitudes toward trainings significantly affected how often they used their wellness training in tutoring sessions.

We asked respondents to identify how often they refer to their wellness training in their tutoring sessions, then analyzed those responses in relationship to their attitudes toward the wellness training they had received. As Figure 1.2 shows, tutors were far more likely to utilize their wellness training during tutoring sessions if they had positive attitudes toward their own training. Furthermore, if tutors did not like the training, they didn't use it more than four times over the course of the semester, which is roughly 1 in 15 sessions.

Furthermore (and this may not be surprising), the more training that tutors receive in center-specific wellness topics, the more their attitudes about homegrown wellness training shifts from low and neutral to positive. Additionally, the more training that tutors receive, the more that they incorporate wellness topics into their tutoring sessions (Figure 1.3). However, three trainings are sufficient for the average tutor to feel positively toward wellness trainings, although tutors seem to use their training more often the more they are trained. In fact, the more training that

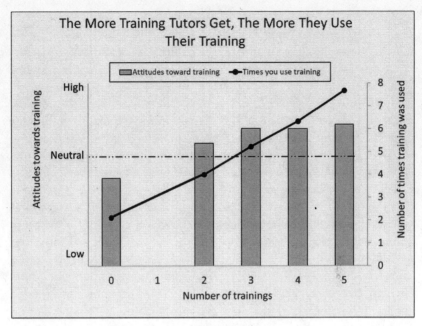

Figure 1.3. The number of wellness training sessions tutors received correlates to the number of times that they used their training. Tutors' attitudes toward training remain fairly consistent and positive after engaging in three or more training sessions.

tutors have, it seems, the more likely they are to report using their wellness training in various aspects of their tutoring practice. This might be because they are incorporating new wellness topics into their tutoring work and doing more cross-referring to services, or it might mean that they are better identifying and reporting wellness work in their tutoring sessions. Either way, findings here indicate that changing the culture of a writing center by implementing wellness training is not met initially with positive feeling by tutors but, over time, tutors come to regard wellness training more favorably and utilize it more in their tutoring work. Training, then, is key to positive outcomes, although I would warn against institutional and workplace wellness programs, as these were not well regarded among tutors (and for good reason) and might lead to low engagement in their tutoring work, as we saw in the initial year and a half of our assessment.

CONCLUSION

I share these findings because wellness interventions in writing center work are not welcomed equally or universally by tutors, often for good reasons. Some tutors mistrust the intervention, others feel anxiety or stress over participating in the intervention, while others simply do not want to think about these matters in relation to writing center work. Some tutors, rightly, are not interested in doing additional work. The legacy of workplace wellness programs in America, as well as empirical findings on these programs, reflect this localized set of issues with both engagement and long-term positive effect on the population, especially in the first couple of years of the wellness training program. In response to these issues with the institutional wellness program, a couple of tutors suggested the center institute an opt-out policy for wellness training, which I agree should be part of any workplace program. Another suggestion they made was to avoid relying on prepackaged wellness trainings (or other university-sponsored trainings) that are disconnected from writing center praxis and everyday experiences. I also agreed with their assessment and totally overhauled our wellness training program to be more consistent with our values, our mission, our staffing demographics, and our work. While institutional wellness programs are a good starting point, insofar as they give us the opportunity to reframe how we engage in our work, these trainings can be, as one respondent noted, a way for the university to dodge their own responsibilities and liability by encouraging self-guided and largely individualistic approaches to wellness. For employees, wellness programs are also bound up with exploitative labor practices and other workplace tensions which, unsurprisingly, tutors are suspicious of and often outright reject. What my tutors and I concluded about institutional wellness programs is that, first, we do not share the values that underpin their philosophy or practices and, second, they are simply not enough—not specific enough, not relevant enough, not interactive enough—to support us in writing center work and other educational spaces.

What I know now but did not when I started on this journey several years ago is that wellness programs are often economically motivated and situated in the individual, rather than the collective. These programs have their genesis in the neoliberal institution and are *imposed* on the individual, and intentionally limited in scope and responsibility to the individual level. This divide-and-conquer approach to wellness is not only cost-effective—and much cheaper to institute than enacting real change in workplace hiring and policy practices—but also a typical kind of approach to controlling labor. Because these programs are vulnerable to distortion by neoliberal politics, it is critical to develop a plan before instituting a wellness initiative. To assess the needs of writing center workers more systematically, but also, more ethically, we ought to, as James and Zoller (2018) advocate, bring employees and management together to co-construct workplace wellness initiatives. This could include creating and disseminating a workplace wellness survey where respondents are asked to identify and order their needs and preferences for support and programming. Another way to do this work is to have small or large group discussions with staff about their wellness needs—Lloyd et al. (2017) provide an example of an employee needs survey (p. 882) as well as discussion questions on wellness needs (p. 884). In the end, however, whatever initiatives are instituted ought to be vetted by writing center stakeholders and, if possible, collaboratively carried out. Instituting these initiatives in a top-down way only roots them further into neoliberal workforce-optimization models, which divorces wellness from its roots in altruistic and revolutionary social movements.

2
UNCOVERING AND ADDRESSING WORKPLACE STRESS IN THE WRITING CENTER

OPENING NARRATIVE

There are many kinds of stressors that one experiences at work. Some might be external to the job but still influence the worker, while others might be internal to the position. Some stressors are punctuated, only occurring once, while others are long-term and occur often. This chapter will share findings on how tutors experience and address different kinds of stress in the writing center. However, I begin this chapter with an in-depth autobiographical account of the active shooter event at Ohio State in fall 2016. I talk about this experience at several points in the book because it was a defining moment for me as an administrator and, also, as a researcher of occupational wellness; yet my findings show that tutors are more concerned with the everyday stressors of their lives and work than they are with punctuated and high stress events.

The Monday after Thanksgiving, it was business as usual at the Ohio State University Writing Center. I arrived around 9 a.m. to open the center and prepare for my mentorship group at 10 a.m. The usual stream of undergraduate and graduate students came in and out of the space. We were in the midst of renovations of various spaces in the center, so the main room that would eventually serve as a lounge for staff and clients was cluttered with unneeded furniture and supplies. Tutors sat perched here and there in that space on desks and chairs that no longer fit in the tutoring rooms.

My weekly mentorship group meeting was about to start. The mentorship group predated me and was a great opportunity to give tutors additional training opportunities during the semester in a small group setting. Eight to ten graduate and undergraduate tutors met weekly to discuss tutoring practices, policies, and, as Chapter 1 discussed, engage in wellness training. One week away from the end of the regular semester, I felt like I had bonded with most tutors in my group.

https://doi.org/10.7330/9781646423606.c002

Before group, I took a quick detour to the restroom. Upon coming out of the stall, a woman I had never seen before told me that there was an active shooter alert, and we were going into lockdown and shelter-in-place. She may have identified herself as the building coordinator, but I really cannot remember.

Living in Cambridge during the Boston Marathon bombing, I was familiar with lockdown and shelter-in-place protocols. In April 2013, the Boston Marathon bombing caused widespread upheaval in Boston and surrounding cities. We were placed under lockdown not once but two or three times during the days following the attack. I was at the marathon before the bombs went off and was biking home during the attack. Four days later, during a shootout between Dzhokhar and Tamerlan Tsarnaev and MIT/Cambridge PD, I was biking back from Central Square—less than a mile away—as a police chase ensued. Reaching further back, I was put under lockdown in high school a number of times following the September 11, 2001, attacks on the World Trade Center and the Pentagon.

I walked quickly back to the Writing Center, silently noting the row of doors that opened from the hallway into our space—a converted physics laboratory with a set of rooms that looked much like a "railroad apartment" in style—a series of rooms in a line with little separation or barriers.

In the center, there were several tutors—those who were getting ready for their next tutoring session, as well as those who were part of my mentorship group. A couple of clients were also waiting for their sessions to begin. In total, there were about 11 students congregating in the cluttered lounge space. I quickly entered and told the group that there was an active shooter on campus, that this was not a drill, and that we needed to lock down the space and shelter in place. We closed the heavy double doors, we closed the doors to the office suite that abutted the lounge, we pulled the shades, we turned off the lights.

In addition to the tutors and students who were already in the center, there were a couple of tutors who were sheltering in place in other rooms in the building. There were also a couple of tutors who were late to mentorship group and were in transit.

Recalling my experiences with bomb threats and gas leaks that caused shutdowns at my previous institution (BCC), I realized that some of the most vulnerable people would be those who were transiting and walking around campus. Immediately, I sent an email to the entire staff urging them not to come to campus and, if they were on campus, to shelter in place. I shared my cell phone number and asked tutors to text me, rather than call, as we had an active shooter alert. As I communicated with my staff, my family and friends tried to communicate with me. News spread very quickly. About 15 minutes after we were given the alert, which was provided through word of mouth to me, I was fielding phone calls, emails, and texts from various family members, colleagues, and friends from around the country. My family told me to barricade the doors. They told me to leave my students. They told me not to be a hero. CNN had reported that there were multiple shooters; so, as I was trying to recall my own experiences, my family was giving advice for sheltering in place that ran counter to university communications or that did not suit specific spaces under lockdown (barricading the doors, for example, might work in some spaces but, in others, it might block the only way out). Proximity to the event had a major effect on the quality of information that we received. In the midst of all of the noise, I had to filter out the panic and the potential misinformation and handle the situation as it was unfolding in front of me, which was hard. It is very difficult to handle a situation on the ground when the media, friends, and family are all reaching out trying to advise from afar.

In the center, I tried to encourage business as usual—not because it was actually business as usual, but because I knew we were in for a long period of waiting while the campus was secured, and I thought activity was a better alternative to just waiting. I asked the tutor whose client had shown up to have their appointment in my office. I promised I would keep watch and inform them if we needed to act. The rest of the tutors in the center listened to news updates through Columbus PD—one tutor, a non-traditionally aged undergraduate student who had been particularly levelheaded during my transition into the directorship—became my second-in-command. Together, we took care of the younger and understandably frightened members of the group. We poured drinks of orange juice and tried to chat calmly. I alternated between spending time with the group and checking in on the tutorial that was happening in my office. I also texted my family and friends and assured them I was OK.

OSU started advising us to "run, hide, fight" fairly quickly after the lockdown and, because of our proximity to the action, we hid. Later, I would learn that many people were unfamiliar with the concept and were unsure of when to run, hide, or fight. Later, I would also learn that we had a knife attack, not an active shooter. In that moment, however, reports about shots being fired and SWAT teams on the roofs of buildings seemed to confirm a worst-case scenario. The attack was at Watts Hall—about a three-minute walk from our building—but misinformation propagated for hours.

In a shelter-in-place or lockdown situation—which are different, I have come to learn—instincts take over, for better and for worse. However, as writing center directors, many of us are not trained to respond to these kinds of punctuated and highly stressful events. The confusion over run, hide, fight; the lack of training about how emergency information is communicated to staff prior to an emergency; the media's intrusion on official university communications; the panic and fear of students and staff—all of this must be parsed and processed in the moment, when an emergency occurs. In Chapter 5, I discuss how to plan for emergencies proactively. But all of that knowledge came later. In the moment, I relied on past experience to guide my actions. No school I had worked for had prepared me for these kinds of events; it was only my previous and personal experience with large-scale emergencies that prepared me to handle this crisis.

One thing I did not learn in my own experiences of crisis, however, was how to process them after the fact. Post-event, restorative practices must be enacted in order to heal. In addition to canceling tutoring for the day following the attack, I also sent out an email assuring the staff that we were going to work on getting through this time together. I reminded them to engage in restorative practices, such as reaching out to friends and family, and taking breaks from work. I reduced the number of people working shifts and worked to accommodate people calling out from work. Around this time, I recognized the importance of allowing tutors the ability to "flex" their hours, especially during traumatic and uncertain times. Framing care work through the dimensions of wellness was useful in developing suggestions for engaging in restorative practices, though I am not sure that I directly referenced them. I also reminded staff of the resources available on campus. Because of these experiences, I later became determined to make wellness interventions—including work policies—an even more substantive element of our training and staff support. But I also became interested in trying to assess and study how wellness interventions and, importantly, stress might impact tutors in their everyday lives—both inside and outside the center.

LITERATURE REVIEW

Occupational Stress—An Overview

Work-related stress is highly researched by a wide-ranging and varied set of local, national, and international agencies, as well as policymakers, businesses, and scholars (Cassar et al., 2020). As Cassar et al. note:

Stress at work, and the phenomena surrounding it, has inevitably gained vast recognition and research attention by various stakeholders and at different levels of society. The phenomenon of work stress has predominantly attracted the attention of policymakers at global, regional, and national levels, scientists across disciplines, organizations across sectors, trade unions, and mass media. (p. 48)

According to the National Institute for Occupational Safety and Health (NIOSH):

Job stress can be defined as the harmful physical and emotional responses that occur when the requirements of the job do not match the capabilities, resources, or needs of the worker. Job stress can lead to poor health and even injury. (NIOSH, 2020)

There is, however, a complex interplay between workplace organization and structure and instances of heightened workplace stress. Sauter (2007), identifies the increasing measures that organizations take to cut costs and outsource labor as heavily contributing to the skyrocketing cases of workplace stress among US workers, which, in 2007, affected one-third of American workers. He notes:

Organizational downsizing and restructuring, dependence on temporary and contractor-supplied labor, and adoption of lean production practices are examples of recent trends that may adversely influence aspects of job design (e.g., work schedules, work load demands, job security) that are associated with the risk of job stress. (Sauter, 2007)

Precarity, in other words, gives rise to increased workplace stress, which affects the mental and physical health of workers, which in turn affects worker performance, rates of chronic illness, and employee turnover. Workplace stress, in other words, heavily contributes to workers experiencing a host of emotional, cognitive, and physical maladies at the same time that these issues contribute to the rising healthcare costs as well as worker-absenteeism and employee turnover.

Both NIOSH and the European Agency for Safety and Health at Work (2020) identify several factors that contribute to work stress. These include:

- Excessive workloads
- Conflicting demands and lack of role clarity
- Lack of agency/autonomy in decision making
- Poor management
- Job insecurity
- Job stagnation—lack of opportunity for growth
- Poor or ineffective communication

- Poor social environment; lack of support from management and/or colleagues
- Poor physical environment; "unpleasant or dangerous physical conditions such as crowding, noise, air pollution, or ergonomic problems"
- Psychological and sexual harassment, third party violence

Stress and Writing Centers

While work stress has been a topic of interest in a number of other helping professions such as healthcare (Ghannam et al., 2020), mental health (Cramer et al., 2020), animal care (Hill et al., 2020), and education (Yu et al., 2015; Arismunandar & Emmiyati, 2016), there is not a lot of research on writing center workers' experiences of work stress or, really, much research on how writing center workers (particularly tutors) perceive their work. Yet many of the identified factors that contribute to work stress are ones that may resonate with writing center workers—particularly those who hold long-term positions that have little growth opportunity.

One early piece (Healy, 1995) that surveyed writing center administrators to better understand how they perceive their work found other work stress indicators—excessive workloads with unclear and conflicting demands—to be heavily present among writing center administrators. In the study, Healy found that WCAs consider work-related stress a moderate job-related issue (p. 32). In the survey, Healy found that "the only significant predictor of job stress was the number of hours per week one spends on writing center work" (p. 35). Other variables, such as staff size, were not accurate predictors of levels of job stress among WCAs (p. 35). Given the large variation in the kinds of jobs writing center administrators perform, "it is very difficult to predict what factors will influence writing center directors' attitudes about their jobs" (p. 35). In Healy's study, he identified a number of frustrations (Table 2.1), which could also be interpreted as work-related stressors, that include a lack of resources (personal and center-wide), a lack of recognition for center work, a rotating and under-trained staff, a lack of defined job duties, and so on. In what is perhaps one of the more comprehensive early studies on how stress-related factors contribute to writing center work, even the articulation of these workplace issues is framed within emotional terms (frustrations) rather than as labor issues (p. 36) or issues of occupational concern.

There are some studies on tutors' experience of work-related stress. Healy (1991) argues that the roles that tutors occupy are at once ambiguous and complex. Studying the professional experiences of tutors

Table 2.1. List of frustrations writing center administrators articulate regarding their work

Work-Related Frustrations WCAs Report	N = 272
Not enough money/staff	66 (24%)
Too many responsibilities, not enough time	45 (16%)
Marginalization of center; lack of recognition and appreciation	42 (15%)
Lack of understanding or support from faculty/administration	41 (15%)
Student and faculty misunderstanding of center's role	36 (13%)
Insufficient facilities, equipment, space	25 (9%)
Finding qualified staff; staff instability, turnover	24 (9%)

Source: Adopted with permission from Healy (1995).

through role conflict "can be helpful in discovering constructive ways to deal with tutorial role ambiguity and conflict" (p. 42). This study acknowledges the reality that peer tutors are not professionalized into the field in explicit ways and that the roles they perform are complicated by the fact that they are vague and lack boundaries. The varied nature of tutoring work causes tutors to experience work stress related to role conflict, which "may result when tutees' expectations conflict with their own preferred style or with their assessment of the best role to adopt in a given tutorial session or at a given tutorial moment" (p. 43). However, in being both peers and tutors, peer tutors also experience role conflict when the many hats they wear as students and employees of an institution bump up against one another. In those clashing moments when role conflict arises, tutors experience work stress. Healy notes that most institutions do not intentionally create stress for student workers; however, he also recognizes the importance of further studying how tutors experience role conflict—and its attendant stress—and to account for it in hiring, training, and mentoring practices (p. 48). We see present in Healy's findings here that work stress may occur among tutors due to excessive and unclear or conflicting demands as well as under-preparation that might result from poor management and/or communication.

Since Healy (1991), others have examined tutors' experience of stress and other attendant negative emotional responses when performing tutoring work or tutor training work (Chandler, 2007). Nicklay (2012) surveyed a tutor population about what prompts them to feel guilt. The findings from the survey included that tutors feel guilty for "betraying the perceived expectations of our center and fellow consultants," such as tutoring in a directive manner (p. 25). Nicklay says these findings are "distressing" (p. 25) because they reveal a cultural undercurrent of distrust in the writing center that runs counter to its attempt to be a collaborative and caring space for its workers. Again, tutors may feel work stress (guilt, in this instance, and fear) due to workplace issues of poor management and communication, but also poor social environment and lack of support.

Implicit within these studies of tutors' experiences of negative emotionality and stress related to their work is a critique of the unclear expectations and practices that underpin tutoring work. For Healy (1991), the unclear and nebulous framing of tutoring work can lead to role conflict when the identities of tutors outside of the center bump up against their identities within the center. For Nicklay (2012), tutoring orthodoxy contributes to tutors' experience of negative emotions while performing their work. Both scholars argue for changes in onboarding and training in writing centers to stave off these kinds of stressors. Nicklay (2012) extends the conversation to include a review of center philosophies as well as how tutoring is conceptualized and enacted (p. 26). Yet there are no studies that examine how job stagnation, job insecurity, and lack of autonomy in decision-making might also give rise to work stress among tutors, although we can surmise from Nicklay's review of tutors' discomfort with working against orthodoxy that they are experiencing work stress related to their feelings of job precarity and lack of autonomy as tutors. Therefore, the complex interplay of work stress ought to be studied specifically as it arises among precarious workers in the field, such as tutors, adjuncts, staff, and other contingent labor that work in writing centers.

Stress is frequently studied from the writer/student perspective, rather than focusing explicitly on the tutor. In "Talking in the Middle: Why Writers Need Writing Tutors," Mickey Harris (1995) explores the tutor's role in reducing stress for writers and enabling them to overcome barriers to learning. Tutors, Harris argues, deal with the affective issues that students experience when writing and, in turn, students benefit from working with tutors insofar as they become more confident, more fluent, and more readily engaged with learning (p. 35). The nonhierarchical structure of peer-to-peer tutorials "relieves strain" and student anxieties (p. 36). In this model, tutors alleviate stress and anxieties while attending to the affective dimensions of the learning and writing processes. However, in our rush to identify the positive outcomes of peer tutoring—it helps student writers (Bruffee, 1984) and it benefits student workers (Harris, 1995; Hughes et al., 2010)—we sideline tutors' experiences of work stress and fail to recognize them as students who *also* experience a range of affective stances in and outside the writing center.

To flip Harris's article on its head, then, we might ask: "What do tutors get out of the experience of working with writers?"

There has been a recent explosion of research on tutor and administrator stress and the attendant anxieties linked to the writing center. Many of these articles focus on mindfulness approaches applied in this context. Mack and Hupp's (2017) "Mindfulness in the Writing Center: A Total Encounter," which was inspirational to my development of a contemplative approach to tutor training (Chapter 4), offers a set of mindfulness interventions (meditation, reflection, loving-kindness, etc.) for tutors to adopt in their everyday tutoring work but also outside the center. Subsequent studies have explored how mindfulness meditation can help to mitigate tutors' experiences of stress during work (Johnson, 2018), while some scholars preemptively anticipate tutor-related stress by creating interventions in tutoring training courses and publishing on their findings; these articles detail supporting pre-professional tutor development and mitigation of stress and anxiety around the practice of tutoring (Featherstone et al., 2019; Emmelhainz, 2020). Still others (Concannon et al., 2020) have extended previous research on mindfulness interventions in tutor professional development instead to administrator professional development. And earlier studies encourage the integration of mindfulness practices, such as meditation and yoga, in writing center work as a way to both reframe tutors' expectations and support tutors in difficult or challenging sessions (Gamache, 2003; Murray, 2003; Spohrer, 2008). A recent study (Simmons et al., 2020) measured the physiological levels of cortisol (stress hormone) on tutors before and after engaging in their tutoring sessions in order to explore what effect tutoring has on stress levels. Except for Simmons et al. (2020), very little research has empirically studied how tutors handle work-related stress and, in particular, the nuances associated with different subtypes and intensity levels of stress, such as extraordinary and ordinary stress. Given the many stressful events that occurred at OSU in the 2016–2017 academic year, I became preoccupied with understanding more about how tutoring might be impacted by experiences of stress, but also what practices might help to mitigate experiences of stress among tutors.

Other research in writing center studies, and attendant fields like composition, focuses on stress not as it relates to labor but as it relates to writing production, composition processes, and writing self-efficacy. Schmidt and Alexander (2012) identify stress as one of the barriers to writing self-efficacy. Their study assessed the effects of a new writing self-efficacy scale on college students that attended the writing center for multiple sessions. There are several other self-efficacy scales that also include stress as one of their metrics (Daly & Miller, 1975; Lavelle, 2010; Bandura, 2006; Piazza & Siebert, 2008). Attendant to writing self-efficacy are the studies on writing apprehension (Daly & Miller, 1975; Atkinson, 2011). Cognitive stress, as Atkinson (2011) notes, may affect the level of writing apprehension a student experiences (p. 5). Each of these studies is writer-focused, so, while research does exist on how writers experience, confront, and avoid stress during the writing process, little research exists on how tutors experience stress in their work with writers. Schmidt and Alexander (2012) study how the writing center can be used as part of an intervention to support student writing self-efficacy, rather than sharing, from a tutor-oriented perspective, how stress might impact their own work.

TUTORS' EXPERIENCES OF STRESS INSIDE AND OUTSIDE OF THE WRITING CENTER

As I briefly mentioned in the previous chapter, once I developed wellness trainings for my writing center staff, I also developed a longitudinal assessment project that measured tutors' experiences of their training and that included a survey with open-ended and Likert scale questions (Appendix B). The survey was administered after each significant revision to the wellness training regimen (2016, 2017, 2018, 2019). Part of that survey also assessed the different kinds of stress that tutors may experience. Included were questions about general coping skills, support structures, engagement with writing center work, management of stress at work, and attitudes toward wellness training initiatives. The survey also sought to answer what, if any, effect wellness trainings had on consultants' behavior during stressful events experienced both inside the writing center (in their work) and outside of the writing center (in their everyday lives), as well as the effect of long-term and short-term stress on tutors. The majority of questions were structured using a Likert scale; however, there were also some ordinal scale questions and open-ended qualitative questions.

I added questions to the survey about how tutors perceive and report handling stressful events because of the high number of stressful events occurring at the time—the 2016 presidential election, "Muslim bans," the rise in hate acts, the knife attack at OSU, the spate of on-campus suicides, the murder of students—which many tutors said impacted them personally. These questions aimed to explain how extraordinary and potentially ever-shifting, stressful events might impact tutors. Questions about extraordinary stress, such as that related to the active shooter

Table 2.2. The Likert scale questions that are related to stress within and outside of the writing center, as well as the codes under which they were calculated and analyzed

---

Coping with stress

I am capable of coping with my daily stress.

I am able to appropriately manage my feelings.

I have positive relationships with colleagues, friends, and/or family members.

I have a colleague, friend, and/or family member I can confide in.

I am confident handling unanticipated stressful events in the WC.

Workplace attitudes

Writing center work gives me a sense of purpose.

The writing center provides me with a community.

My job at the writing center produces stress in my life.

I am comfortable communicating with colleagues at the writing center.

I am comfortable communicating with clients at the writing center.

The writing center cares about my well-being.

The writing center provides a positive work environment for me.

Current events stress

How much have you been concerned by the knife attack on campus?

How much have you been concerned by the presidential election and current administration?

How much have you been affected by the death of OSU students (Reagan Tokes, Heather Campbell/recent suicides on campus)?

How much have you been affected by the posting of racist and anti-diversity flyers?

---

alert, the presidential election, and other campus and national events were amended each year. I also recognized, drawing from Degner et al.'s work on tutors' long-term experiences with mental health concerns (2015), that ordinary stressors might also contribute to tutors' everyday lives and their workplace habits and experiences. Therefore, I also included more general questions about tutors' daily stress levels, their social support, and their engagement with writing center work. From the group of questions that asked about various levels of tutor stress and workplace expectations, I created several codes including:

1. Coping with stress score
2. Workplace attitudes score
3. Current events score

The questions listed in Table 2.2 were combined to develop each of these codes.

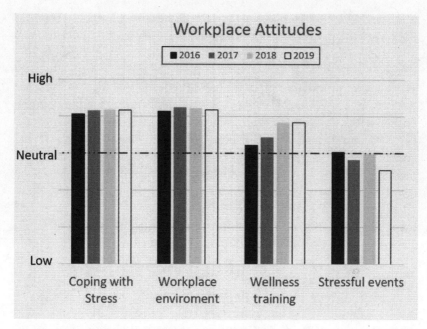

Figure 2.1. Tutor workplace attitudes, including attitudes about their personal abilities to cope with stress; their attitudes toward the Writing Center and their work; their attitudes toward wellness training; and their attitudes toward stressful events occurring outside the writing center.

FINDINGS

As one can surmise from the codes, I was interested in how tutors experience stress both inside and outside of the Writing Center, as well as whether their experiences of stress affect their attitudes toward their writing center work. I was also interested in how tutors rank their coping with stress skills. Work stress, as I came to realize from reviewing survey findings, is much more elusive to track than attitudes toward wellness training. Most tutors reported very positive experiences in the Writing Center workplace as well as high confidence in their coping skills (Figure 2.1). Tutors' confidence in their coping skills included positive and high confidence in their abilities to handle stressful events, their support networks, and their management of feelings. Although at first I thought that tutors would have a variety of coping skills—and this may lead to better or worse coping with stress—this was not the case. Similarly, I thought that attitudes toward the workplace might also impact their ability to cope with stress, but here, too, they reported very consistent attitudes toward the Writing Center. Similarly, after we changed our wellness training, tutors also reported higher and more consistent confidence in that element of writing center work. In short, my statistical analysis for the coping with stress scores and the tutor workplace attitudes scores did not have any significant variation. These scores showed tutors with largely positive attitudes toward the Writing Center as a workplace and in their abilities to navigate stressful situations within the Writing Center and their personal lives.

Yet, tutors' reported attitudes toward stress external to the Writing Center tells us a slightly different story about how they perceive stress. Here, we see tutors rating their attitudes toward stressful events in generally neutral to negative ways (Figure 2.1). This suggests that tutors might be unlikely—because of varying factors related to job security—to articulate negative feelings about their workplace and their coping skills. However, stressful events that are external to the writing center are, perhaps, considered safer to report feeling concerned about.

Not all tutors are affected by stress in the same ways, however (Figure 2.2). While undergraduate and graduate tutors both reported nonsignificant and little to no concern over short-term stressors such as the active shooter alert and student deaths, graduate tutors reported significantly higher concern than undergraduate tutors regarding long-term stressors, such as those related to the presidential election and consistent alt-right broadcasting through racist, anti-Semitic, anti-immigrant fliers on campus. 2018 in particular, which was the midterm elections in the United States, seemed to be a high mark in the graduate students' reportage of relatively high concern over these events. This suggests that the year in which the tutor responded to the survey contributed to their attitudes about stressful events.

Of course, I assumed that punctuated stressful events—such as the active shooter—would profoundly contribute to tutors' reportage of high stress levels; however, as it turns out, undergraduate tutors reported relatively low concern regarding any stressor, and graduate tutors reported high but varying concern about long-term stressors. This suggests that different populations in the Writing Center might interact with external stressors in different ways or might discount stressors outside of the Writing Center as not impacting their work; therefore, it is critical to not only assess but also address different kinds of stress among different populations. As a WCA, I was terrifyingly concerned about the active shooter situation (short-term stressor), likely because I experienced it not only as an individual but as someone responsible for a group of vulnerable people. While my staff seems generally unconcerned about this issue, it is perhaps because many tutors did not experience this situation in the same way that I did. Of course, risk and emergency management, and how to behave during an active aggressor

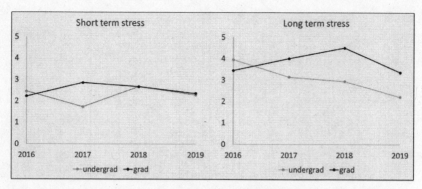

Figure 2.2. How undergraduate and graduate tutors are affected by short-term and long-term stress by year, with graduate tutors feeling significantly different, and more concerned, about long-term stressors in 2018 than undergraduates. Tutors are not concerned as much by short-term stress, with a nonsignificant difference between undergraduate and graduate tutors in their low rating of concern about short-term stress.

situation, became a significant part of our wellness training following the active shooter on campus; therefore, concern over short-term stressors like this might have been low among the tutor population because of these factors. Still, I continue to think about short-term and long-term stressors and assess how tutors feel and perceive different kinds of stress to get insight into training and discussion topics.

CONCLUSION—ADDRESSING WORK STRESS IN THE WRITING CENTER

Of course, my interest in stress only scratched the surface of the kinds of stressors that tutors may experience in doing their work. While I was focused on what one might call extraordinary stressors, tutors would come to me every day with relatively ordinary stressors that I took for granted as being part of writing center work. Eventually, I came to realize that because tutors are all coming into the Writing Center with different experiences and traumas, these ordinary stressors might actually contribute far more to the work stress that tutors experience than a stray gas leak or fire emergency. So, there is much more to do in terms of unpacking the different kinds of stressors that tutors experience and how they cope with them. More research needs to be done to assess what kinds of work stress tutors experience in the Writing Center. As I demonstrated above, findings also suggest that asking directly in a survey about tutors' satisfaction with the Writing Center as a workplace might not yield honest (or at least varied) findings.

Table 2.3. Actions WCAs can take to mitigate specific work stressors

Workplace Stressor	Action Items
Excessive workloads	Set clear limits on workloads and review them regularly with workers.
Conflicting demands/lack of role clarity	Set clear workplace expectations and review them regularly with workers.
Lack of autonomy in decision making	Welcome worker input and feedback; implement nonhierarchical decision-making processes for selected policies and initiatives.
Poor management	Act according to the values and goals you set for your center; lead by example; develop a workplace culture that values individual workers.
Job insecurity	Advocate for long-term positions such as tenure track WCA and assistant WCA positions; advocate for salary increases and job security for hourly workers.
Job stagnation	Offer workers opportunities for professional development and growth—attending conferences, developing and running center-wide trainings, conducting research, publishing.
Poor or ineffective communication	Create a communication plan and stick to it; develop training and policy documents that are readable and accessible.
Poor social environment	Set workplace expectations for peer-to-peer and WCA support; create community through shared activities, trainings, and goals; recognize and reward workers' job performance.
Poor physical environment	Contact ergonomic/occupational wellness departments on campus to do a site visit—conduct your own site assessment to mitigate "hazards" in the workplace.
Psychological and sexual harassment, third party violence	Require Title IX training; set and discuss workplace policies on micro- and macroaggressions; require implicit bias and antiracist trainings.

Surveys, then, might not be the first step in assessing how tutors experience work stress. In fact, policy enactment and discussion might be more useful here in order to lay the groundwork for conducting more robust and in-depth research on work stress. There are many different policies that might address work stress in our field. I start with advocating for increased job security and setting workplace standards that are non-exploitative but, also, that help individual workers thrive. This is no easy task, especially given the recent and recurring crises in higher education that many of us are facing. However, there are some ways to address work stress that start at the local level and that include ways to develop a strong workplace culture that is anti-racist, positive, aware of individuals, and non-coercive/exploitative (Table 2.3). Some interventions include providing tutors with professional development and leadership opportunities, pay raises, manageable workloads, and clear workplace expectations through training, documentation, and mentorship. Additionally, and new as of the pandemic, our center has started setting aside time for non-training-based community building activities such as tutor meetups and processing events. Investing in tutors, especially student tutors and adjunct/staff tutors, is critical to mitigating some of the work stress that arises out of precarious, overly taxing, and ambiguous work.

3

CONDUCTING WELLNESS RESEARCH AND ASSESSMENT IN WRITING CENTERS

OPENING NARRATIVE

While searching for institutional and field-specific information on workplace wellness and mitigation of stress, I realized that there was little empirical research that specifically examined the occupational experiences of student workers in higher education. In writing centers, the research on tutors' experiences of work is bracketed into very distinct and narrow topics related to writing center-specific labor such as tutoring work—adhering to orthodoxy (Nicklay, 2012)—or factors that render tutors unable to perform their tutoring work, such as mental health concerns (Degner et al., 2015). Except for studies such as that of Simmons et al. (2020) and a more recently published chapter on cortisol and physiological stress (Nelson et al., 2020), we know little about how tutors experience stress while on the job. There are, in other words, a complex set of phenomena—some within the control of the WCD and some outside of our control—that affect tutors' engagement with their work and retention in the writing center. I was interested in a broad array of internal and external factors that may affect tutors' work, such as how tutors experience and cope with stress. I was also interested, as Chapter 1 demonstrates, in how tutors' occupational experience of the writing center is shaped by their training and support in wellness topics.

So, in addition to researching institutional wellness programs, such as the one offered by my institution on positive psychology, and learning about occupational stress and how it impacts workers' experience of their jobs, I also created a wellness-focused survey for student workers in the Writing Center. As I discussed in the previous two chapters—and I will continue to discuss throughout this book—findings from my workplace wellness assessment profoundly impacted how the Writing Center supported worker and workplace wellness through enacting new policies and interventions. Here, I provide a primer for those interested in

https://doi.org/10.7330/9781646423606.c003

conducting similar research in their own centers (or other educational workplace sites). This chapter moves from general best practices for conducting research to more detailed guidelines for how to work with wellness data using quantitative and qualitative approaches. Along the way, I use my research project—and some key findings—as a model to discuss specific elements of study design, data processing, and data analysis. The second half of the chapter is fairly technical as it shares details from statistical analysis that were found using RStudio, an analysis program that uses the coding language R. In that section, I provide examples from my own dataset as models for discussing nonsignificant and significant findings and what these might mean for one's project outcomes. But first, some background on wellness research and study design.

BACKGROUND

There are many ways to do research on wellness in writing centers. In a chapter in the digital edited collection *Wellness and Care in Writing Center Work* (Giaimo, 2021), I give an overview of the different methods that scholars in our field utilize to conduct research on wellness topics. The top three methods are:

- Survey
- Interview
- Artifact collection of reflective writing (session notes, student reflections, journal entries, etc.)

There are, however, many other ways to study and measure the effect of wellness interventions on different populations. One interesting approach is that of biological sampling through minimally invasive methods such as saliva collection to measure tutors' cortisol (stress hormone) levels before and after engaging in tutoring work (Simmons et al., 2020). Another is the inclusion of autobiography and personal experiences related to issues of wellness and labor that also include storying (Green, 2018).

Wellness research tends to share some similarities, such as that studies predominately focus on writing center workers (tutors, WCAs, tutors-in-training) rather than writing center clients, few studies have clearly articulated methods and study participant numbers, and, when articulated, the sample sizes for empirical research on wellness often include a small number of study participants. Because a lot of the research on wellness in writing centers focuses on writing center workers—rather than clients—it makes sense that sampling sizes are low. Small research populations still tell us a lot about tutors; namely, in this instance, how they engage with wellness training interventions.

ON WORKING WITH SMALL DATASETS

Because of the growing popularity of "big data" in writing studies, researchers might be apprehensive to develop a study that only captures a small subset of a population or a small population. Different researchers address this cohort issue in different ways. Degner et al. (2015), for example, administered their survey on mental health concerns to tutors through an electronic listserv. I chose to administer the survey to a single research site (OSU), because of its specific engagement with the wellness training intervention; therefore, I elected to do a longitudinal design in which I administered the survey four times over the course of 3.5 years. Taking into consideration the average population size of the OSU Writing Center ($n = 48$) and the response rate ($n = 64$), as well as the percentage of staff changeover between years (25%), I calculated that the response rate for this survey was roughly 50% of the potential respondent population, which is much higher than the usual 20% rate that researchers aim to secure in their survey work.

There are many reasons why this research—especially on tutor populations—will be small. One of these is the fact that writing centers often contain relatively small numbers of staff. Therefore, researchers might want to include a longitudinal component in the study design, especially if a survey instrument is utilized; however, researchers may elect to collect other kinds of data such as tutor observations, tutor interviews, tutor focus groups, artifact collection, etc. In a previously published article of mine (Giaimo et al., 2018), for example, I collected and analyzed a year's worth of tutor session notes ($n = 7,000$) utilizing corpus linguistic analysis and Voyant, an open access text analysis tool, to identify keyness—terms used with significant frequency in a given corpus—for specific terms tutors utilized to describe their work. What I found is that tutors often talk about "help" when describing their work but, digging down into the collocates, or phrases often associated with these words, I found that tutors were mostly talking about their *inability* to help their clients, rather than their ability to do so. From this and other linguistic analysis on that dataset, I recognized that tutors are doing a lot of emotional labor in their tutoring work that needed to be addressed. There are many methodological approaches, then, to studying questions related to wellness and labor.

Because of my background in psychology, I am interested in empirical ways to study how tutors, rather than clients, engage with wellness; therefore, my research work naturally turns to experimental design. For the study that produced the data in this book, I settled upon a mixed methods survey administered multiple times to the OSU tutoring staff from 2016 to 2019 (Appendix B). The survey and the training models (Appendix A and Appendix C) were developed in tandem and informed one another.

DEVELOPING THE EXPERIMENTAL DESIGN

Before undertaking any research or assessment of wellness, I thought about the experimental design for my study. First, I identified the population I wanted to assess, which, in this case, was tutors, and what I wanted to learn from studying them, which, in this case, was how tutors engage with wellness training. Then, I thought about a number of variables that might affect tutors' engagement with wellness training, which included factors that ranged from the demographic (tutors' rank, tutors' semesters of WC experience, the year in which the training and assessment were provided), to the attitudinal (tutors' ability to cope with stress, tutors' attitudes toward current stressful events, tutors' attitudes toward working in the Writing Center, tutors' evaluation of the wellness trainings) to the behavioral (tutors' reported number of wellness training engagements, tutors' reported utilization of wellness training). From here, I developed a number of hypotheses about what I thought I would find in assessing tutors' perception of and engagement with wellness training, as well as their confidence in handling stressful events. Some of these hypotheses included the following:

- Hypothesis 1: Tutors' ability to cope with stress affects their engagement with wellness training.
- Hypothesis 2: Tutors' attitudes about their jobs affect their engagement with wellness training.
- Hypothesis 3 (more specific): Tutors who have fewer coping skills and who experience more stress related to their writing center work are less likely to engage with wellness training in a positive way.

Some Best Practices for Experimental Design Include the Following:
- **Develop your study with an eye toward replication.** Indeed, this might be one of the most important elements to experimental design, which is to say that the method, materials, participation selection process, and analysis are all clearly articulated and able to be replicated by others. One fun exercise I do with my students

is to ask them to develop a "research protocol" for making coffee. Usually, students forget to include a critical step, such as adding water or coffee grounds to the pot. In giving a simple "how-to," students are able to better understand both the specificity and detail with which methods are produced. Starting with experimental design that maps these elements out is critical to securing human subjects research approval from one's Institutional Review Board; it also helps researchers to stay on track during data collection and produce clearly articulated methods in publication format.

- **Consider a baseline set of data or a control group within study design.** Many educational studies include control groups that do not receive an intervention (pedagogical or otherwise); however, there are ethical considerations in limiting access to what might ultimately be a positive intervention. Therefore, another way to do this work is to see where cohorts form in naturally occurring ways (i.e., within and among groups who do not have equal access to an intervention). In my study, I included longitudinal surveying to collect a baseline in the first year of the intervention (where it was novel and less curated than in subsequent years), which helped me to identify the change in respondent attitudes, over time.

- **Identify any variables that might confound your results, such as evaluation apprehension or social desirability effect.** These can later be "blocked" out of analysis by identifying them in analysis as "nuisance" variables. Confounds are more important, I would argue, in more controlled experimental design such as ones that you might see in a laboratory setting or in experimental design that includes educational datasets (here, I am thinking about performance metrics) that are relatively large and contain a number of variables. In wellness research, which is often carried out in naturally occurring settings with quasi-experimental design, there might be few cofounding variables, or the confounding variables might indeed be of interest to the researchers.

- **Randomize data collection, if possible.** This can be achieved through randomized participant selection, though when studying a relatively small population (tutors at a specific writing center), randomization might not be possible. In this case, identifying the threshold response rate (20%–25% is typical)—the minimum number of respondents that still represents your population—is critical to the study's validity. Furthermore, developing a survey that might eventually be disseminated outside of your writing center can help the researcher to further randomize data collection and get data from a larger sample size.

DEVELOPING THE SURVEY

I developed the questions in the survey (Appendix B) to include demographic questions, behavioral questions, attitudinal questions, and perceptual questions. Attitudinal and perceptual questions were grouped and coded under "domains" that measured respondents' engagement with wellness. Some of these domains, such as the coping with stress domain, asked about respondents' lives outside of the Writing Center, while others, such as the workplace attitudes domain, asked about respondents' experiences within the Writing Center. Because of my interest in studying perceptions, and because of a number of hypotheses that posited how tutors' engagement with the wellness trainings is influenced by circumstances external to the Writing Center (such as personal attitudes about coping with stress), I took a multipronged approach to measuring tutor engagement with wellness that also asked about tutor habits, attitudes, and experiences around this topic.

So, in developing the various domains—and attendant research questions—related to topics about wellness, I also had to ask questions about where tutors were coming from in terms of their experiences with stress and their attitudes toward stressful events occurring nationally and around OSU. These questions formed the basis of my study design as well as my survey instrument.

Some Best Practices for Developing Survey Questions Include the Following:
- Avoid asking questions that might identify individual study participants.
- Avoid asking questions that might cause undue harm or stress on study participants.
- Avoid asking questions that have multiple questions or parts.
- Ask questions in different registers/tones—negative, neutral, positive.
- Include questions in the survey that function as control questions. For example, in the current events stress domain section, a question was included in the survey about anti-Trump fliers on campus alongside questions about racist fliers posted on campus and DACA and visa bans. The anti-Trump question—not included in final coding—was included as a control question to determine if respondents were answering the survey in good faith and answering consistently. If respondents are concerned about both anti-diversity flyers and anti-Trump fliers, depending on their other responses, it is likely they are not answering the survey in good faith. If, however, they are concerned by anti-Trump fliers but unconcerned by anti-diversity fliers, visa bans, DACA uncertainty etc., they are likely answering the survey in good faith. Any survey responses that did not answer in good faith were excluded from final analysis.
- In developing questions, account for multiple rounds of surveying. For example, some of the questions in the current events stress

domain changed from year to year in response to recent events
occurring at the national and local levels.

- Phrase questions in such a way that they offer a range of response
  (Likert) rather than dichotomous (yes/no) responses.

- Include open-ended responses—in addition to Likert scale
  questions—that offer nuance and depth of response.

- Ensure Likert scale questions (strongly disagree–strongly agree) are
  arranged consistently on either a 5-point or 7-point scale and that
  they share similar language for response (and that the language fits
  the question's phrasing).

- Ensure that questions have a similar linguistic structure, and be prepared to rescale responses to questions that are phrased in the negative, for example, when coding data.

- Prepare Likert scale questions in an order that allows for creating
  codes rather than analyzing single responses. Likert scale responses
  are typically nonparametric, which means they do not have a normal distribution among the 5- or 7-point scale (just think about
  responses to student evaluations that fall out at the far ends of
  strongly agree and disagree). Therefore, in developing questions in
  groupings or domains (Table 3.1), the researcher ensures easier data
  processing, which includes moving single questions into grouped
  codes that are closer to a normal distribution curve (and therefore
  parametric). The kind of distribution affects the kinds of statistical
  analysis one can perform on their data.

A BRIEF HISTORY OF RESEARCH ETHICS AND ITS
IMPLICATIONS FOR WELLNESS RESEARCH

Although it is a requirement of most American educational institutions
that researchers undergo human subjects training and submit research
proposals to an institutional review board (IRB) before undertaking
any research on human subjects, there are factors beyond institutional
regulations that one should consider before engaging in such research.
Throughout history, and within our lifetime, there have been numerous
studies with questionable or outright unethical design and egregious
treatment of subject participants. Some of these, such as the Tuskegee
syphilis study, treated their subjects so egregiously, that they led to governmental intervention and major reform of human-subject research
protocols. The Tuskegee syphilis study, which was run from 1932 to 1972,
recruited Black men from rural areas to study the effects of syphilis.
The researchers withheld diagnosis from the study participants as well
as treatment for syphilis, even after penicillin became a standard part of
course of treatment in the 1950s (Kim, 2012, p. 5). After congressional
hearings, the National Act, which created the National Commission

Table 3.1. Domains and survey questions included in each scored domain

Coping with stress
I am capable of coping with my daily stress.
I am able to appropriately manage my feelings.
I have positive relationships with colleagues, friends, and/or family members.
I have a colleague, friend, and/or family member I can confide in.
I am confident handling unanticipated stressful events in the WC.

Workplace attitudes
Writing center work gives me a sense of purpose.
The Writing Center provides me with a community.
My job at the Writing Center produces stress in my life.
I am comfortable communicating with colleagues at the Writing Center.
I am comfortable communicating with clients at the Writing Center.
The Writing Center cares about my well-being.
The Writing Center provides a positive work environment for me.

Current events stress
How much have you been concerned by the knife attack on campus?
How much have you been concerned by the presidential election and current administration?
How much have you been affected by the death of OSU student (Reagan Tokes, Heather Campbell/recent suicides on campus)?
How much have you been affected by the posting of racist and anti-diversity flyers?

Wellness Training Score
My wellness training has prepared me to handle stressful events in the Writing Center.
My wellness training has helped me to support colleagues at the Writing Center.
My wellness training has helped me to support clients at the Writing Center.
The wellness training prompted me to develop new methods of helping others at the Writing Center.
Wellness training changed the ways in which I handle stressful situations beyond the university setting.
Wellness training has changed the ways in which I would respond to university-wide emergencies.
A culture of wellness matters to our work at the Writing Center.

for the Protection of Human Subjects of Biomedical and Behavioral Research, was passed in 1974. The commission published the Belmont Report in 1979, which provided a set of ethical principles for conducting human research (p. 5).

The three guiding principles developed from the Belmont Report are:

- Respect for persons
- Beneficence
- Justice

These principles protect peoples' autonomy through developing an informed consent process in which the purpose, benefits, and potential risks of a study are articulated in plain and understandable terms. Researchers must be truthful to study participants, give them the option to withdraw from the study, and, importantly, can "do no harm" to participants. Engaging in research that is nonexploitative and administered fairly and equally from the development of experimental design, study participant protocols, through carrying out study procedures and interventions, aims to ensure that studies like Tuskegee—where rural Black men did not receive diagnosis and treatment for a curable and debilitating disease—do not happen again. The Belmont Report is a cornerstone of IRB policies and regulations and heavily informs IRB proposals developed by researchers (Kim, 2012, p. 5).

When considering ethics, one might assume that educational research—especially when compared to medical research—has little chance of harming subject participants. In fact, even in other fields, such as medicine, it might be difficult to anticipate the risk of conducting research on human subjects: "Protecting human participants in research is our top priority and has been given great consideration in the ethical conduct of research because the exact risks and benefits of research are uncertain" (Kim, 2012, p. 3). Before undertaking any kind of research related to whether people engage in wellness practices, or about their experiences with stress and wellness, it is critical to consider the very real benefits and risks of studying this topic. Some risks that I considered prior to developing my research study included asking questions that might trigger a traumatic memory related to OSU's lockdown and/or the deaths of students. Another risk I considered was that in answering questions about habits around stress and wellness, tutors would realize they have less support in their lives than they need and/or they are less equipped to handle stressors that arise in and outside the Writing Center. Some benefits that this study might produce included tutors who were more trained in handling stressful events in the Writing Center, tutors who were able to draw from a larger repository of activities to manage stress and engage in care, and tutors who made beneficial changes to how they engaged with stressful aspects of their lives (such as coursework). Ultimately, some of these benefits were reported in the open-ended responses in the study.

When developing a study on tutor wellness, or wellness among clients/writing center administrators, consider the following:

- What are the (most likely to least likely) risks to engaging with my research study?
- What are the (most likely to least likely) benefits to engaging with my research study?
- What kinds of support does my institution have if respondents need mental health support?
- How am I going to report out findings from my study?
- How am I going to represent research participants in my research?
- How can I include human subjects in my study beyond collecting data from them?

Because a lot of educational research and assessment can benefit curricula, professionalization and training programs, and the general outcomes of programs such as the Writing Center, there is a lot of good that can come from conducting human-subject research in such settings. However, there is also a responsibility that researchers have to their research participants to ethically engage them in the research process, which includes faithful and "thick" representations of findings. As the Conference on College Composition and Communication (CCCC) statement (2015) on research ethics suggests, researchers should report any qualitative data "in ways consistent with the collected data, and [that] avoid deliberately misrepresenting participants' words." The statement suggests providing context for participants' words, as well as consulting with participants if there are any doubts about intended meaning. Such steps are even more crucial if study participants are not made anonymous.

A NOTE ON NEGATIVE RESPONSES

It is OK to have respondents reflect negatively on their experiences in surveys. In fact, negative responses are as informative—or perhaps even more informative—than positive responses! From survey responses, I found that tutors reported relatively positively and consistently, over time, on the coping with stress domain, as well as the workplace attitudes domain. However, as I noted in Chapter 1, respondents significantly varied in their response to the wellness training with far more negative responses occurring in 2016 and 2017 and far more positive responses occurring in 2018 and 2019. This suggests that a change took place in tutors' attitudes toward wellness training over the years, which makes sense because the training was also significantly changed—based on tutor feedback—throughout that time.

Table 3.2. Example of data processing and coding approach for abbreviated versions of responses to questions related to coping with stress domain

ID	Rank	Survey Year	Semesters of WC Work	I cope with my daily stress	I manage my feelings	I have positive relationships	I can confide in	I am confident handling unanticipated stressful events in the WC	Score
1	Grad	2016	3	4	4	3	4	4	3.8

HOW TO PROCESS THE DATA

To process responses, I create a CSV file (Excel) to code the data. Respondents and their responses are included on the row and individual questions and their codes are included on the column (Table 3.2).

Once all data is coded, I review the dataset for unfaithful responses (again, reviewing all control responses), gaps in responses, and incomplete responses. I then remove any respondents that did not complete the survey or who did not respond to the survey in good faith.

Once the numerical data is coded and all Likert scale questions are included in a scored response, I then import the data into RStudio.

At this point, I consider my variables—independent or predictor variables (tutor ID, rank, survey year, semesters of experience, etc.) and dependent variables (coping with stress score, workplace attitudes score, current events stress score, wellness training attitudes score, etc.) and build a linear model that will analyze an independent variable against its dependent variables. For the purposes of the data shared in this book, I conducted a three-way ANOVA (analysis of variance) on a number of variables from the dataset.

CONDUCTING ANALYSIS

I used the programming language R, which, while specialized, also has a vast array of free online resources on how to utilize it for statistical analysis. The RStudio website (rstudio.com) has a number of cheat sheets, tutorials, and code banks that are free to use. Below, I share the code for my statistical analysis along with ANOVA for specific variables in order to discuss select nonsignificant and significant findings.

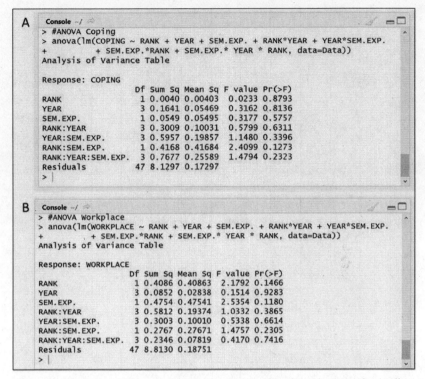

```
A   Console ~/
    > #ANOVA Coping
    > anova(lm(COPING ~ RANK + YEAR + SEM.EXP. + RANK*YEAR + YEAR*SEM.EXP.
    +            + SEM.EXP.*RANK + SEM.EXP.* YEAR * RANK, data=Data))
    Analysis of Variance Table

    Response: COPING
                        Df Sum Sq Mean Sq F value Pr(>F)
    RANK                 1 0.0040 0.00403  0.0233 0.8793
    YEAR                 3 0.1641 0.05469  0.3162 0.8136
    SEM.EXP.             1 0.0549 0.05495  0.3177 0.5757
    RANK:YEAR            3 0.3009 0.10031  0.5799 0.6311
    YEAR:SEM.EXP.        3 0.5957 0.19857  1.1480 0.3396
    RANK:SEM.EXP.        1 0.4168 0.41684  2.4099 0.1273
    RANK:YEAR:SEM.EXP.   3 0.7677 0.25589  1.4794 0.2323
    Residuals           47 8.1297 0.17297
    >
```

```
B   Console ~/
    > #ANOVA Workplace
    > anova(lm(WORKPLACE ~ RANK + YEAR + SEM.EXP. + RANK*YEAR + YEAR*SEM.EXP.
    +            + SEM.EXP.*RANK + SEM.EXP.* YEAR * RANK, data=Data))
    Analysis of Variance Table

    Response: WORKPLACE
                        Df Sum Sq Mean Sq F value Pr(>F)
    RANK                 1 0.4086 0.40863  2.1792 0.1466
    YEAR                 3 0.0852 0.02838  0.1514 0.9283
    SEM.EXP.             1 0.4754 0.47541  2.5354 0.1180
    RANK:YEAR            3 0.5812 0.19374  1.0332 0.3865
    YEAR:SEM.EXP.        3 0.3003 0.10010  0.5338 0.6614
    RANK:SEM.EXP.        1 0.2767 0.27671  1.4757 0.2305
    RANK:YEAR:SEM.EXP.   3 0.2346 0.07819  0.4170 0.7416
    Residuals           47 8.8130 0.18751
    >
```

Figure 3.1. Results from three-way analysis of variance in RStudio with no significant effects by year, rank, or semesters of experience on respondents' confidence in their ability to cope with stress (A) and their attitudes toward the writing center workplace (B).

Interpreting Findings: Nonsignificant

While findings that are significant (results not attributed to chance) are important to deriving meaning from the dataset, so too are findings that are not significant, where no change is measured, or changes measured are due to chance (the null hypothesis) (Canning, 2014). To explain why having nonsignificant findings can still help us derive meaning from our data, I return to some of the variables that I discussed in Chapter 2 (Figures 5 and 6): the workplace attitudes domain and the coping with stress domain, respectively. Here I share my statistical analysis, represented by the output from the R code, that shows no significant effects of year, rank, or semesters experience on either workplace attitudes or coping with stress (Figure 3.1).

As I noted previously, several of my hypotheses regarding how tutors engaged with wellness training revolved around how they coped with stress inside and outside of the Writing Center, as well as their attitudes about the work in the Writing Center. Upon conducting my analysis on these variables, however, I found that students were overwhelmingly positive about both their ability to cope with stress and their views on the Writing Center as a workplace. The average coping score was 4.14 (sd ± 0.41), with the lowest coping score being 3, which represents a neutral response. Likewise, attitudes about Writing Center work were overwhelmingly positive with an average response of 4.19 (sd ± 0.42), with the lowest workplace score being 2.71 (slightly negative) and the highest score being 4.86 (highly positive).

There are many reasons why statistical tests are not significant—namely, there is not enough variation in respondents' responses—however, I can surmise from these findings that there is little variation among respondents in terms of how they reported on their ability to cope with stress as well as their attitudes about the Writing Center workplace. In both domains, tutors reported quite positively. Therefore, in trying to figure out how tutors engage with wellness training—such as if there are factors that limit their engagement or affect their attitudes toward workplace wellness programs—I found that their reported ability to cope with stress (which was, again, quite positive) and their attitudes about writing center work (also quite positive) did not have a measurable effect on how they perceive or engage with wellness training.

Observing no difference among groups, however, isn't bad or a failure in a research study. In fact, it indicates that there might be some regularities (or biases) among the study cohort, which tells me that directly asking tutors about their ability to cope with stress, or their satisfaction with the workplace culture of the Writing Center, are, perhaps, not the best ways to elicit genuine responses. Or perhaps tutors are satisfied with the workplace culture of the Writing Center and, at the moment of their response to the survey, confident that they can cope with stress. Or perhaps satisfaction with workplace culture does affect how tutors engage with workplace wellness training. Such nonsignificant findings, then, are an invitation to ask more detailed questions that look deeper into specific areas where we might measure some divergence among groups within the study population.

Interpreting Findings: Significant

There are instances in conducting statistical analysis, however, where the null hypothesis can be rejected in favor of the alternative hypothesis, which is that the factors being investigated have an effect on one's variable of interest (p value) but, also, the order of magnitude of the effect

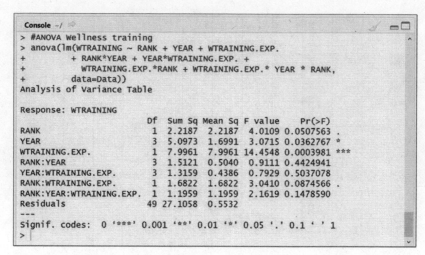

```
Console ~/
> #ANOVA Wellness training
> anova(lm(WTRAINING ~ RANK + YEAR + WTRAINING.EXP.
+            + RANK*YEAR + YEAR*WTRAINING.EXP. +
+              WTRAINING.EXP.*RANK + WTRAINING.EXP.* YEAR * RANK,
+        data=Data))
Analysis of Variance Table

Response: WTRAINING
                         Df  Sum Sq Mean Sq  F value    Pr(>F)
RANK                      1  2.2187  2.2187   4.0109 0.0507563 .
YEAR                     3  5.0973  1.6991   3.0715 0.0362767 *
WTRAINING.EXP.           1  7.9961  7.9961  14.4548 0.0003981 ***
RANK:YEAR                3  1.5121  0.5040   0.9111 0.4424941
YEAR:WTRAINING.EXP.      3  1.3159  0.4386   0.7929 0.5037078
RANK:WTRAINING.EXP.      1  1.6822  1.6822   3.0410 0.0874566 .
RANK:YEAR:WTRAINING.EXP. 1  1.1959  1.1959   2.1619 0.1478590
Residuals               49 27.1058  0.5532
---
Signif. codes:  0 '***' 0.001 '**' 0.01 '*' 0.05 '.' 0.1 ' ' 1
>
```

Figure 3.2. Results from three-way analysis of variance in RStudio with significant effects by year and wellness training experience on respondents' attitudes toward their wellness training.

(effect size, F score). For example, in this study there is a significant and large effect of year (F 1,64 = 3.07, p = 0.036) and a significant and large effect of number of wellness trainings (F 1,64 =14.45, p < 0.001) on tutors' attitudes toward wellness training (Figure 3.2). This suggests, as I discuss in Chapter 1, that respondents respond to wellness training differently in surveys that they take in different years. We see this interaction in Figure 1.1 with respondents in 2016 and 2017 responding more negatively regarding their wellness training than respondents in 2018 and 2019. The other significant finding with a large effect size, also discussed in Chapter 1 (Figure 1.3), is that the number of wellness trainings that tutors receive strongly affects their attitudes toward wellness training. The more trainings tutors engage in, the more likely they are to have positive views of wellness trainings. These findings are reproduced in the raw output from RStudio in Figure 3.2.

Over time, tutors become more engaged with wellness training and are more likely to respond to it favorably in later semesters of engagement than in earlier semesters of engagement. This makes sense for several reasons, namely that there was a lot of resistance to wellness training when it was initially introduced to the staff, and, in their open-ended responses, respondents reported less favorable engagement with institutional wellness training than with homegrown wellness trainings that were offered in later semesters in the Writing Center. The year that the tutors received wellness training as well as the number of wellness trainings they receive, then, are predictors of their attitudes toward workplace wellness training. Significant findings, then, help us to figure out what effect, if any, changing workplace wellness trainings has on tutors' engagement with these interventions.

CODING OPEN-ENDED RESPONSES

Open-ended questions allow respondents to engage with more nuance than they can to questions with scaled responses. Therefore, inclusion of open-ended—qualitative—questions are critical for diving deeper into the attitudes, perceptions, and behaviors of survey respondents. We included a number of open-ended responses in the survey, including:

- What strategies have you developed in identifying wellness needs in others? Please elaborate or provide an example.
- Can you share an episode or event, within or outside of the Writing Center that allowed you to use any wellness training skills developed from Writing Center training?
- What recommendations would you give for future wellness training opportunities?

Of course, the third question enables continuous engagement with the training intervention and allows the training model to be part of a more iterative process. Relying upon subject input for feedback helps to:

1. Identify any gaps in the training intervention as it is currently conceived.
2. Further develop the training intervention over time.

Experimental models—and the interventions they enact—need not be stable. In fact, when creating and carrying out a longitudinal survey, it makes sense to introduce additional design elements and then to measure their efficacy as compared with the other interventions. Having baseline data is critical to such measurement of change in attitudes and perceptions over time.

The open-ended responses could be coded several different ways, such as by keyword frequency, by topic, by tone/affect (positive, negative, neutral), or by other kinds of linguistic and/or thematic groupings. For the purposes of this study, qualitative findings were included in the discussion to offer nuanced and more deeply articulated attitudes about wellness training. As many of the individual responses show, there were deep and sometimes conflicting responses to wellness training, even after we switched over from an institutional wellness program to a bespoke, in-house one; therefore, providing text-based responses (preferably in their entirety) lends insight into how tutors think critically about wellness training and its place within the Writing Center and in their lives more broadly. I also included raw count numbers for topical occurrence (such as responses that indicated uptake of mindfulness strategies in tutors' personal lives) to highlight similarities across responses.

VISUALIZING DATA

There are also many ways to visualize data. For publication purposes, it is critical that any publications include tables that show the results of the statistical analysis, including significance, sum of squares, degrees of freedom, and other elements commonly reported utilizing APA standards (2020). Not only is this important information that informs the validity of findings but it also paves the way for future researchers to conduct additional statistical tests, such as meta-analysis, on a corpus of empirical studies centered upon a similar topic, such as wellness.

In addition to tables, figures are also critical to visualizing significance for readers, especially in the field of writing studies, where readers might not be able to understand a table with details from a statistical analysis quickly or easily. While line graphs are useful and relatively easy for visualizing two to four variables, more sophisticated visualizations include models such as PCA (principal components analysis), which shows grouped variables in relation to one another, as well as heatmaps, which are useful in showing individual variation/frequency within and among cohorts of participants. For more information on data visualization, review Mueller's (2017) *Network Sense: Methods for Visualizing a Discipline*, the special issue of *Kairos* recently published on visualizing data in composition studies, and "A Periodic Table of Data Visualization" (n.d.) for ideas and examples of different kinds of visual representation of data.

HELPFUL RESOURCES FOR STUDY
DEVELOPMENT AND DATA ANALYSIS

There are many fine examples of books in writing center studies, as well as in the larger field of writing studies, that detail the research process from study design and enacting data collection procedures to analyzing and reporting out findings (Babcock & Thonus, 2012; Kinkead, 2015; McKinney, 2015; Ianetta & Fitzgerald, 2016; Mackiewicz & Babcock, 2019). However, for statistical analysis support, I really enjoy John Canning's *Statistics for the Humanities* text, which is open-access and quite readable.

CONCLUSION

In this chapter, I advocate for planning and designing an intentional and ethical research study. At the same time, I also recognize the important role that serendipity plays in many elements of the research process. Research in our field is different than empirical research in the sciences. For example, one may do post-hoc analysis on data that has already been collected in order to determine the most effective statistical analysis, rather than identifying and sticking to the same analytical approach at the outset of a study. And, of course, unlike research in a laboratory setting, there are often variables, or circumstances, that we cannot control or might not want to control. These kind of natural experiments—ones occurring "in the wild," so to speak, are filled with complexities but, also, with exciting possibilities. The purpose of this research, then, is not to carry it out in perfect conditions, or to rigidly follow a protocol and approach without deviation but, rather, to bring intentionality to the planning and implementation stages of the research process. With some planning and forethought, research studies can be carried out with more ease but also with attention to elements like ethics that help the researcher not to run afoul of the IRB and potentially cause harm to study participants. Therefore, under most circumstances, if a research study on wellness is being planned, IRB approval needs to be secured—retroactive approval, particularly for this kind of research, should be sought only in the most unique and limited of circumstances (think, here, about research that includes artifact collection or other kinds of data collected from people who have left the institution) and should not be the default, especially for novice researchers.

In studying wellness and other habits related to the attitudes, emotions, and behaviors of tutors, first think about harm and benefit to research. Consult with colleagues. Share sample survey and interview questions. Run a pilot of the study and amend accordingly. Like most cognitive processes, research is not static or linear. However, it can be intentionally planned and carried out. Of course, an interest in wellness suggests that the researcher is likely hoping to improve conditions for their study participants or learn something novel about their participants to apply that knowledge to the field; therefore, the study design ought to account for motivations as well as potential outcomes from data collection.

We owe it to writing center practitioners to engage in this work in ethical and sustainable ways. This means avoiding coercing people into participation and, also, recognizing when the intervention might not be working, as I experienced with the first wellness training program that was provided by the institution. For me, the wellness study revealed how our intervention both met and did not meet tutors' needs. From our findings, we adjusted the intervention accordingly, but I also came to a lot of personal realizations about how wellness support and training might simply not be enough to support tutors and that we must also look to policy changes alongside any center-specific interventions.

WHAT COMES NEXT?

The first section of this book has argued that wellness interventions that are corporatized and enact bootstrap rhetoric are problematic, but also, even localized and bespoke wellness interventions are not enough; any intervention needs to be paired with top-down action such as the enactment of policies that recognize and reward labor, offer flexible work policies and fair wages, and that are safety-focused, inclusive, and anti-racist. Wellness work must be comprehensive and addressed at several structural levels from the institution on down to center administrators and individual workers. Findings from my research showed me that tutors' workplace feelings, attitudes, and behaviors about work are not just about the workplace itself but about the complex factors that they face both inside and outside of their job. Just as external stressors can affect workplace culture and sentiment, so too can workers' sense of their safety within broader institutional and national contexts. So, while perceptions of workplace culture matters (and ought to be assessed), a complex set of factors outside of the job (and our control) have profound effects on workplace satisfaction, engagement, turnover, and performance. Neoliberal practices that have been adopted by university workplaces, such as inflexible leave policies, low wages, and different kinds of physical and material precarity hurt us and our staff.

At the same time, we struggle to get out from under the neoliberal practices adopted by university workplaces without being given encouragement, guidance, training, and, yes, permission. Correctives to the neoliberal workplace, then, are complex, multifaceted, and rooted in policy as much as practice. In the chapters that follow, I offer several wellness correctives that rely on both policy and practice. Chapter 4 provides mindfulness training interventions alongside fairer labor policies. Chapter 5 provides workplace emergency planning policies alongside post-trauma processing activities. Chapter 6 provides resources to combat burnout caused from emotional labor alongside policies to mitigate these workplace experiences. And Chapter 7 resituates wellness work in community and self-care practices, anti-racist activism, and Black feminism alongside offering policies on how to do anti-racist wellness work in the writing center. These chapters are correctives to what I see as the relatively hollow and apolitical valences with which wellness interventions (mindfulness and self-care practices) and wellness issues (be they physical or emotional) are framed in much of the current research in our field. By rooting wellness in anti-materialist, anti-racist, and anti-exploitative theory and research, I hope we can build complex networks of workplace wellness practices and policies that are restorative and rooted in well-being rather than labor optimization and other neo-liberal goals.

PART II

Finding Wellness Interventions that Work

4

INCORPORATING MINDFULNESS INTO INTENTIONAL TUTORING PRACTICE AND POLICY

OPENING NARRATIVE

The crises that occurred in 2016—particularly the active shooter situation detailed in Chapter 2 and its aftermath, which I discuss in Chapter 5—but also other local crises like the deaths of OSU students and national crises such as the revocation of DACA and the Trump travel bans all affected my decision to make mindfulness the theme of the 2017–2018 academic year. As with the previous year's theme on wellness, I was excited to integrate some of the newly published mindfulness interventions into our Writing Center. At this time, several tutors—including graduate coordinators—also indicated interest in mindfulness interventions in the center. By the end of the year, however, we recognized that mindfulness practices, while important, need to be shored up with labor policies that similarly prioritize tutor wellness over labor outcomes.

Mack and Hupp's (2017) article, "Mindfulness in the Writing Center: A Total Encounter," which had been published the previous spring, was influential in our incorporation of mindfulness exercises into tutoring training. Some of the graduate student coordinators and I developed mindfulness exercises to complement the mentorship group training schedule for the fall semester (Appendix C). Mentorship groups met weekly for an hour and included anywhere from eight to ten tutor participants and one facilitator. The groups included training topics with mindfulness activities. Some activities (such as pairing a breathing exercise with a repetitive drawing activity, called "breathing lines") were gleaned from a yoga retreat that I attended. Others, such as mindful appreciation, were created by individual graduate student coordinators. Because graduate coordinators and I each led mentorship groups (there were anywhere from four to six groups per semester, depending on staff size), we co-trained and discussed these activities as a group before we implemented them and then reflected on their impact and success afterward.

https://doi.org/10.7330/9781646423606.c004

The mentorship groups were an ideal place to implement the mindfulness activities. For my part, I hoped that inclusion of mindfulness exercises would support the following goals:

1. Create community formation among tutor cohorts.

2. Positively guide discussions about stress and other feelings related to writing center work.

3. Shore up some of the work policies that we instituted.

4. Create intentionality and reflection around tutoring practice.

Upon my arrival at OSU, there were several great professional development practices in place, such as pre-semester training workshops and the weekly required mentorship groups. But, because the Writing Center was largely run by graduate coordinators, the mentorship groups lacked consistency and focus. Each group spent its time differently and these hour-long weekly meetings were not consistently used for training purposes. Instead, they often devolved into "complaining sessions" about tutoring work. Many peer and graduate tutors expressed their discomfort with this model and also questioned the efficacy of these groups. In the first year, I aimed to add more consistency across the groups—I developed a weekly discussion topic schedule (that looks a lot like a syllabus)—and I added specific training elements and professional development elements to weekly meetings with the group facilitators. Part of this work focused on wellness, such as the three-week wellness training workshops that were facilitated by university wellness ambassadors.

In year two, mindfulness activities were added to the mentorship group schedule. Previously there had been little done to discuss stressful events—internal or external to the Writing Center—in productive ways. Most emergency meetings were held in response to events that had already happened, which meant that we could never seem to get ahead of stressors in our work or contemplate a different way forward in engaging with them. Additionally, if no crises occurred, the meetings focused on the more mundane elements of tutoring, such as connecting with library services. My turn to mindfulness methods, then, was proactive in the sense that my experiences as an administrator were teaching me the importance of pre-training tutors in different responses to crises and stressors. However, I was also hearing from tutors that they wanted more meaningful support and training to do their work. Mindfulness, I felt, helped to address several needs I saw in the center, and among the staff.

Most mindfulness interventions in writing centers are incorporated through training—whether inside the writing center or embedded within a tutor training course—and often include several opportunities for staff to engage in these activities. Mack and Hupp (2017) introduce the concept of mindfulness to their staff in a themed retreat and then establish a set of weekly mindfulness activities in which tutors are encouraged to engage. Featherstone et al. (2019) include mindfulness meditation in their tutor training course in order to sharpen students' metacognitive focus in preparation for tutoring work. Emmelhainz (2020) includes guided meditation in her tutor training course in order to prepare and train students for their tutor role. Mindfulness has been found to help tutors-in-training to negotiate anxieties around the act of tutoring and to develop their skills in observation and being "non-judgmental" (p. 2). Concannon et al. (2020) utilize mindfulness practices to train graduate and faculty administrators in developing their mentorship skills. Johnson (2018) advocates for the inclusion of mindfulness meditation into writing center practices for tutors and students alike "as a stress-reducing strategy" (p. 24). Mindfulness practices, then, are bound with labor practices, whether they are incorporated into training to allay anxieties over tutoring, to encourage skill-building in areas such as metacognition, active listening, and observation, or to "potentialize writing center tutors' supportive roles," as the title of Johnson's (2018) piece articulates.

I would be remiss if I did not also acknowledge the ways in which I hoped mindfulness would meaningfully and positively affect the workplace culture of our Writing Center. We faced several challenges related to team-building and cohort-forming ranging from staff size (55+ tutors), to physical location (there are seven physical and online sites), to the previous administrative model in which graduate students did most of the center's day-to-day work. These challenges were compounded by our space limitations—our main center could comfortably hold five or six tutorials at once—which contributed to our previously inconsistent approach to staff-wide training and professional development. Mindfulness activities helped to establish a different and more coherent culture in our Writing Center while also helping tutors to connect with each other and with themselves through a kind of collective routine.

LITERATURE REVIEW

The Origins of Mindfulness and Its Adaptation to American Contexts

Mindfulness interventions in the United States were largely popularized by Jon Kabat-Zinn, a professor emeritus of medicine at UMass Medical Center. Zinn established the Center for Mindfulness in

Medicine, Health Care, and Society at the University of Massachusetts Medical Center as well as the Stress Reduction Clinic. He "developed and began conducting mindfulness-based stress reduction (MBSR) in 1979" (Huxter, 2015, p. 29). Kabat-Zinn defines mindfulness as "moment-to-moment, non-judgmental awareness, cultivated by paying attention in a specific way, that is, in the present moment, and as non-reactively, as non-judgmentally, and as openheartedly as possible" (2015, p. 1487). His work on mindfulness extends back decades and has been influential in the medical field and, more currently, the field of neuroscience. Zinn's research focuses on how mindfulness interventions can be used in clinical practices, such as to mitigate experiences of stress (Kabat-Zinn, 2003), chronic pain (Kabat-Zinn et al., 1987), and other health issues. His work has been incredibly influential across a number of fields that study mindfulness, in addition to mindfulness-based stress reduction, dialectical behavior therapy, acceptance and commitment therapy, and mindfulness-based cognitive therapy (Huxter, 2015).

Since Kabat-Zinn, mindfulness interventions have been adopted in a wide array of contexts, such as in business (Bartlett et al., 2019), health professions (Westphal et al., 2015), law enforcement (Fisher et al., 2019), education (Roeser et al., 2013; Sun et al., 2019; Klingbeil & Renshaw, 2018; Tarrasch, 2019), activism (Gorski, 2015), writing centers (Mack & Hupp, 2017; Johnson, 2018; Featherstone et al., 2019; Emmelhainz, 2020; Concannon et al., 2020), and in the broader field of composition (Kroll, 2008; Harrison, 2012; Wenger, 2015; Consilio & Kennedy, 2019), including writing program administration (Wenger, 2014; Moore, 2018). Much of the research on mindfulness cites stress, burnout, and other adverse effects from engaging in professional work—as well as experiencing workplace stress—as impetuses for implementing and/or examining how mindfulness might mitigate these adverse and work-related experiences. Some studies, particularly those in the field of education (Roeser et al., 2013; Sun et al., 2019; Klingbeil & Renshaw, 2018; Tarrasch, 2019), make explicit reference to occupational stressors, such as burnout, and the need for more teacher training that addresses worker welfare.

While the language that Kabat-Zinn, and many scholars, utilize to describe mindfulness is detached from its Buddhist roots (Maex, 2011), the concept was, nevertheless, heavily guided and influenced by Zen Buddhism and the teachings of Thích Nhất Hạnh (Kabat-Zinn, 2011). To that point, mindfulness extends much further back than four decades; its antecedents in Asian philosophy are well over two millennia old. Grounded in Buddhist teachings, mindfulness is profoundly connected to and contextualized by Buddhism's Noble Eightfold Path (Huxter, 2015). While modern-day secular definitions of mindfulness often rely on being aware in a non-judgmental way, Buddhist definitions of mindfulness also include acts of remembering (*sati*) and clear comprehension or introspection (*sampajanya*), which, ultimately, can lead to wisdom (*punya*), which can be defined as "reason, logic, and intuitive knowing" (p. 32). Mindfulness, as Huxter (2015) notes, is connected to other behaviors beyond "bare attention" (*manasikara*) (p. 31): "From a Buddhist perspective, skillful mindfulness cannot be separated from the context of wise discernment and acting in accordance with principles of harmlessness, which are integral aspects of the Buddha's the eightfold path leading to awakening" (p. 32).

The eightfold path is "a way to balance any imbalances of connotation, attention, cognition, and affect" (p. 33). Through a number of sub-systems, it offers an interconnected framework "that inhibits or uproots the types of mental, emotional, and behavioral patterns that cause and perpetuate psychological suffering" (p. 33). It promotes the development of "optimal, compassionate, and wise ways of perceiving, being, and understanding" (p. 33). I quote heavily here from Huxter (2015) to drive home the point that the origins of mindfulness in Buddhist teachings have not been fully examined in many fields that utilize mindfulness practices, including in writing center studies. The mindfulness interventions that are described by Huxter are not shallow or insubstantial; they involve a persistent and regular amount of remembering, introspection, and ethical engagement. They are, in many senses, therapeutic and transformative. It is important to consider the ethical ramifications of asking our staffs to engage in mindfulness work, especially as, through doing so, it might unearth traumatic or otherwise complicated memories and experiences.

MINDFULNESS IN WRITING CENTERS

While a lot of the research on mindfulness revolves around workplace stress, and the attendant issues that are connected to being part of a "helping profession," broadly defined, writing centers have not fully examined the origins of non-Western mindfulness practices nor the impact of implementing mindfulness interventions in writing centers. At the same time, however, mindfulness has become increasingly referenced as a training approach for tutors. Most mindfulness research in writing centers focuses on training and paraprofessional initiatives, which suggests that our field is converging on a shared theory that our tutors (and graduate administrators) are underprepared for the work that they perform and need support in developing skills that are critical to those in the helping professions. However, while mindfulness is often presented as a "value-neutral" wellness strategy, Ratnayake (2019) suggests that "mindfulness follows the trend for simplicity and individuation. Its embedded assumptions about the self make it particularly prone to neglecting broader considerations, since they allow for no notion of individuals as enmeshed in and affected by society at large" (2019). To extend Ratnayake's argument to our field, little has been written on broad and systemic issues among writing center workers such as burnout and other occupational stressors, yet there is a lot of research on wellness interventions as a way to better prepare tutors for their work. And, in some cases, as with Johnson's (2018) piece on mindfulness meditation and tutor preparation, a focus on optimization of tutor labor through mindfulness interventions is both acknowledged and welcomed. Mindfulness, in this instance, is a tool that helps management to further capitalize on already at-risk and contingent labor through coercive training programs marketed as skill-building.

This wellness model does not examine *why* mindfulness is a necessary corrective in writing centers and other educational spaces. Instead, it responds to the exigency with little forethought. Of course, burnout from emotional labor and other wellness issues impact tutors in the center. For good reason, then, mindfulness interventions are increasingly being included in tutor training and professional development. Yet framing these interventions, as much of our research does, on preparing tutors for such wellness issues rather than examining the systemic issues that create these issues in the first place doesn't do justice to answering why mindfulness interventions are a growing and central element of tutor professional development programs. Even Mack and Hupp (2017), with their focus on professional tutors, use veiled language of labor optimization when describing the success of their mindfulness intervention: "100 percent of the consultants who participated in the poll claimed that incorporating mindfulness practices into the writing center had a positive effect on student consultations" (p. 13). In this instance, Mack and Hupp frame customer—rather than worker—satisfaction as one of the main positive outcomes of the mindfulness intervention. They frame this work as positively affecting outcomes rather than substantively contributing to workplace culture or a more ethical model of writing center labor. Little thought seems to be given to why professional tutors, specifically, might feel lowered empathy or fatigue from their tutoring work.

In this mode, mindfulness interventions are incorporated into writing centers to produce better laborers, not happier or more satisfied or less precarious tutors. In many instances, the connection between tutor preparation and mindfulness ignores how the rhetoric of wellness is coopted unconsciously to solve a problem that may be a smokescreen for the actual problem; that is, to produce better workplace outcomes rather than produce better workplaces. Administrators might fail to recognize that we are making these rhetorical moves when we incorporate such wellness interventions into our centers because we may believe that we are simply preparing our tutors for their jobs or, perhaps more insidiously, protecting them from the negative experiences of their work.

Yet in failing to parse the individual from the institution, or the cause from the symptom, we lean into these neoliberal figurations of workplace wellness programs and use them to shape our programs and our staff. And we rely on mindfulness research that is largely divorced from its Buddhist (and anti-capitalist) origins, instead implementing interventions bound up in neoliberal thinking about workplace outcomes and tutor performance. Monty (2019) identifies this shift toward more commercially minded approaches to our work as one influenced by the

> neoliberal academy, where institutions of higher education assume, a narrow, economistic and market-oriented understanding of "utility" and "relevance" . . . [and] a *de-academization of knowledge* . . . "characterized by the entry of the university into marketplace relationships and by the use of market strategies in university decision making." (p. 37)

In this model, the mindfulness interventions that we provide our tutors become an extension of the neoliberal academy and create better labor outcomes and "profit margins" rather than protecting or otherwise supporting individual tutors or improving actual workplace culture. Therefore, WCAs ought to scrutinize *why* mindfulness is being incorporated into the writing center at higher rates—for "humanitarian or educational benefits" or, conversely, as a "return on investment" in tutor labor (p. 37).

WELLNESS PROGRAM ASSESSMENT FINDINGS

Even as I critique the very real pitfalls of incorporating mindfulness in writing center work, I also recognize that mindfulness activities can be very popular with tutors and administrators alike. Throughout the last 3 years of the survey, tutors regularly reflected on how the mentorship group mindfulness activities impacted their personal and professional practices. Several respondents ($n = 15$) reported that they had begun to incorporate mindfulness practices into their everyday lives, such as in engaging with friends and family, developing study habits, or working through their own feelings. One respondent noted: "I used the mindfulness training during my midterms because I will feel overwhelmed with responsibilities and I find it very helpful to destress via the tips learned at mindfulness training." Another wrote: "After the mentorship wellness training where we took 5 mins to write down everything that was stressing us out and everything we had to do, I've gotten in the habit of doing it almost every week."

Several respondents ($n = 24$) also reported incorporating mindfulness strategies into their tutoring sessions between 2017 and 2019. As many other scholars (Mack and Hupp, 2017; Featherstone et al., 2019) have noted, and my survey also found, tutors reported that mindfulness practices helped them to destress between sessions. They also developed pedagogies that incorporated mindfulness activities into their tutoring sessions. One respondent wrote in 2017 that their training affected their ability to "listen and feel compassion for the clients. When my client told me that she felt stressful about her schoolwork, I told her that feeling stressful is normal and many people feel the same way as she did. At the same time, I asked her to tell me about it." Another respondent wrote in 2017: "A mindful approach to sessions allows me to remain open to the subtle cues of wellness needs that clients may offer during consultation. I often find my clients opening-up about stress and specific life challenges they face day to day at OSU simply because I open myself up to really hear them." Such responses demonstrate tutors engaging with compassion and "loving kindness" in order to better understand and guide their clients.

Another respondent in 2018 noted that while mindfulness activities might have not been popular generally with the staff, they enjoyed engaging with mindfulness because they had prior knowledge and experience with such practices. They note: "The most frequently used wellness skill I have used is mindfulness. I practiced mindfulness long before I came to the WC, but I did learn new techniques in mentorship that I enjoy, such as the lines drawn on paper. I enjoyed those activities, although I know most people did not."

Another tutor wrote in 2019 about how mindfulness helped them to engage in emotional management and self-talk more effectively:

> I think I have mostly used wellness training skills in how I talk to myself. This past year has been emotionally and physically draining for me personally, and strategies like mindfulness help me ground myself when I feel like I need a recharge. I specifically try to use practices of gratitude in my mindfulness to change my thinking from negative to positive. For

example, this morning I woke up feeling exhausted to my bones, but I knew I had to lead mentorship which is important to me and to the consultants in my group. I tried to refocus my thinking from "I am exhausted" to "I am thankful I have enough energy to do what I need to do." It helped a little (as did coffee!).

Of course, what is lurking in this response and similar ones is the ways in which mindfulness activities and trainings fall short of fully supporting tutors. In many ways, this comes out most clearly here in terms of the respondent trying to shift negative feelings about workplace duties and expectations to positive ones. While this tutor, who identifies as a leader in the writing center, seems to effectively utilize their mindfulness training, this negotiation between personal feelings and workplace responsibility indicates that workplace expectations need to be amended to account for workers' feelings of burnout and exhaustion. The hazard of mindfulness strategies, like other wellness trainings, is that they place profound expectations upon practitioners to perform in ways that *seem* mindful but might be, in reality, deleterious to such an enterprise.

I will say, however, that an unanticipated finding that came out of the assessment of our wellness training is how many tutors adapted mindfulness strategies and activities into their personal lives. More than any other training that we provided, mindfulness training deeply impacted tutors in their lives outside the Writing Center. This suggests that we need to better prepare student workers (or, perhaps, just students full stop) for negotiating the stress of college life. Since incorporating this kind of wellness training into the Writing Center, I have also added it to my tutor training course and my 100-level writing course. Contemplative writing practices are a popular area of research in composition (Wenger, 2015; Kinane, 2019), and students as well as faculty seem to favorably respond to these approaches in the classroom (Barbezat & Bush, 2013). Therefore, while these strategies might be useful in helping tutors develop some of the skills they need to engage in tutorials, mindfulness strategies can also play an important role in students' development of skills outside of a writing center context.

The purpose of this book is to help colleagues who want to implement wellness training and support into their programs to avoid neoliberal versions of these interventions that focus more on workplace outcomes than individual success or engagement. Wellness interventions, then, should benefit tutors and clients as much as or even more than the institution's financial incentives or optimization of a program's outcomes. At OSU, as at most other institutions, we invested in mindfulness interventions for tutors to support them in their day-to-day work.

It was my hope that the occupational stressors of tutoring work, such as burnout, reduced empathy, and heightened negative emotions would be reduced by creating a culture of care around writing center work. In other words, I used mindfulness work, in part, to help tutors connect with the pleasure and positive experiences of their work while also hoping they could reflect upon and manage the negative experiences of their work. Tutors, I realized, need spaces to both engage with and critique their tutoring work. They also need permission, it seems, to slow down and take breaks.

What I learned from this intervention is that we cannot rely on wellness as the only corrective for workplace issues. We also need to move away from unrealistic and inflexible work policies, especially for our student workers and our adjunct workers, and make space for tutors to talk about their negative feelings in addition to their positive ones about writing center work. This is perhaps my one major concern with mindfulness training, that it can be coercive insofar as many of the activities encourage practitioners to practice gratitude and "loving kindness," which can feed into a toxic positivity culture. Therefore, I suggest making mindfulness practices optional rather than compulsory. I also suggest opening with examining or critiquing some of the mindfulness activities such as asking what tutors think the place of gratitude and loving kindness ought to be in a workplace. Additionally, as I argue elsewhere and reiterate here, we need more than wellness training if we want to develop ethical labor sites that not only protect workers but also empower them to feel a range of complex emotions about their work, and about writing centers more generally. To that end, tutors and I drafted several labor policies that we hoped would complement and shore up our center's mindfulness training and support models and address experiences of worker fatigue and burnout.

Our Revised Labor Policies Included:
- **Flexing contract hours**: Graduate student tutors could move or "flex" their weekly hours between different weeks of the semester, at their discretion.
- **Sick time**: We reviewed our sick time policies and, in concert with HR and the graduate school, revamped our sick time policies to include a set number of hours that were included in short-term sick leave.
- **Long-term leave**: We reviewed university, local, state, and federal sick leave policies and developed an articulated long-term family and medical leave policy.

- **Shift coverage**: We stopped relying on single tutors in our smaller sites, both for security purposes and so that tutors felt empowered to call out.

- **Remote work**: We offered reliable synchronous and asynchronous online tutoring to allow tutors who needed more flexibility in their schedules different work options.

- **Scheduling**: We no longer allowed tutors to schedule most or all of their hours in single shifts (which could range from 4 to 8 hours in a day!) We also instituted a mandatory break in between blocked shifts of more than 3 hours.

- **Payment**: I asked HR to conduct an assessment of undergraduate student hourly payment across the university to determine if we could give undergraduate tutors a raise*

  * Unfortunately, HR never pursued the undergraduate wage assessment initiative; however, wage equity is an initiative I have brought to my current institution and one that I encourage WCAs to advocate for.

CONCLUSION: MORE THAN MINDFULNESS

As the findings from my assessment on workplace wellness interventions show, institutional wellness programs often fail to provide meaningful and positive change in workplaces because, in many ways, these programs were designed to optimize and streamline labor. At the same time, mindfulness interventions developed in-house can impact tutors in professional and personal contexts. Center-specific training and supportive work such as regular mindfulness practices can lead to positive engagement with workplace wellness. Workplace policies that place material and physical wellness front and center in the workplace's culture and values system are important to shore up such mindfulness practices. Further wellness interventions, then, include top-down interventions such as the labor policies discussed here alongside compensated mindfulness interventions. In Chapter 7, I will discuss further development of this work to include intersectional, collective, and deliberately anti-racist activist approaches to workplace wellness. In Chapter 5, I discuss emergency planning and crisis response best practices and policy templates that will help center administrators plan for emergencies, train their workers, and, post-crisis, process trauma (an action that is notably absent from many institutional emergency plans and protocols). Taken together, these policies and approaches articulate, in a way I am unsure wellness trainings can do, an anti-neoliberal figuration of writing center work.

5
EMERGENCY PLANNING AND RISK ASSESSMENT IN THE WRITING CENTER

OPENING NARRATIVE

Ohio State's directive to shelter in place during the active shooter alert was not the first, or even the second, time that I have experienced a large-scale school shutdown and shelter-in-place event. I've lived in two different cities that experienced terrorist attacks that caused the cities to issue shelter-in-place and lockdown orders. I saw firsthand how such unexpected and profoundly public attacks can lead to all kinds of issues including misinformation, panic, and, afterward, PTSD. So, when, less than four months into my new position at OSU, a building coordinator said that shots had been fired next door to the Writing Center and the area was under lockdown, I was not necessarily ready, but I was at least familiar with many of the protocols in place to handle such situations. Most people have less experience than I did with these large-scale emergencies but, as Kaitlin Clinnin (2020) rightly identifies in her chapter on the 2017 Las Vegas shooting, we are living in an age of widespread crises, "the frequency of crisis events suggests that it is no longer a matter of if a crisis will occur but a matter of when" (p. 130). Clinnin's experience in several active shooter events that occurred in different parts of the country—as well as my own experience with mass crises—shows us that we need to better train and prepare for emergencies that previous generations of educators might have never encountered. As writing center administrators, we do a lot of training; emergency and risk management planning and crisis response should matter just as much as topics related to writing center praxis.

Emergency and risk management is a difficult area for many writing center administrators to get their heads around. Often, it involves planning for the worst while calculating the likelihood that any one particular disaster will occur. Is the campus more likely to experience a shooting event or a knife attack or a tornado or a hurricane? Understanding

https://doi.org/10.7330/9781646423606.c005

one's local context such as the climate, gun laws, crime demographics, and student populations, might help to guide preparation for the least and most likely campus-wide emergencies. But, as several current studies and stories centered on the pandemic (Kvatum, 2020) note, humans are particularly bad at calculating risk.

And risk assessment doesn't happen in a vacuum; it is affected by personal feelings and experiences as well as those of the people around us such as family, friends, and colleagues. A lot of the misinformation and potentially dangerous events that occurred during OSU's lockdown deeply affected me. I had family calling me and urging me to get off campus during the lockdown, while I was coordinating and calming more than a dozen tutors and clients in two different parts of the Writing Center that were not physically connected. Tutors emailed and asked whether they should still come to campus for their shifts. Tutors were locked out of the Writing Center, but, also, in other areas of the building, because they did not understand what shelter-in-place meant and they hid in open-area lounge spaces. So, what started as a mundane Monday morning—during which many consultants were coming or going for various purposes—very quickly turned into a logistically complex emergency with little forewarning. I had to weigh each potential request using my own complicated comfort with risk.

After the lockdown, I realized that we were missing a clear emergency protocol, which is why I relied so heavily on my prior experiences with crisis management. While the university had recommendations for developing building emergency plans, it was not until this crisis came and went that I found out we had such a plan for the building that houses the main site of the Writing Center. In the version of the plan published online at the time, the Writing Center was not even included among the occupants of the building plan although we had been in the building for five years at that point. In other words, the building's emergency plan failed to include us even though we occupied a large part of the fourth floor and had a satellite site on the first floor of the building. I also received no training on emergency management or risk assessment on a college campus. At that point, I didn't know whether inclement weather or a terrorist attack was more likely to occur. I call attention to what we were missing at OSU in the hope that it will help other writing center administrators to be more proactive in getting the information they need to do their jobs as safely as possible during emergencies.

Part of this work includes more training—or at least information—on risk assessment. One of my first acts as director of the OSU WC was to circulate the active shooter video developed at the university. I came of age during the Columbine High School shooting and felt that active shooter training was critical in an educational setting. Although there was still a lot of confusion about how to shelter in place and what exactly "run, hide, fight" meant, I am sure that this addressed at least some of the surface questions about handling a campus-wide shooting event. Of course, this is just one of several possible emergencies that we educators may face in our work. And, as the COVID-19 pandemic has taught us, some of these crises may be less likely but far more devastating. But the larger issue, as I experienced it at Ohio State, was one of communicating expectations. It is not enough to load templates, videos, and emergency plans onto websites and hope that faculty and staff take up the charge to do such work. We need explicit training and support to develop, carry out, and assess our emergency plans.

The rest of this chapter focuses on the history of emergency planning in higher education and how to build an emergency plan and do crisis response work. While the literature review below provides a primer on this field and articulates how institutions of higher education assess risk and plan for and respond to emergencies, little research in emergency planning talks about the ethical dimensions of this work. Student workers are often left out of crisis response, for example. Emergency plans are often not anti-racist and inclusive but instead rely on law enforcement without considering how people of color might be affected by such a plan. And, finally, supportive practices in the post-emergency phase are often left out of emergency plans in higher education, which minimizes the wellbeing of our communities for the sake of "carrying on." Given these oversights, I go into more detail about how to develop an emergency plan in an educational setting such as a writing center (Appendix D) that considers these critical factors. Planning in an emergency, I suggest, should involve all departmental stakeholders (WCAs, tutors, perhaps even clients) and should also involve any emergency planning teams and safety professionals on campus. It should, however, also consider inclusion, safety, and wellbeing for all community members.

LITERATURE REVIEW

A Brief History of Risk Assessment and Emergency Planning in the United States

While risk assessment and communication can be traced back to before Greco-Roman civilizations, when the ancient Babylonians used "myths, metaphors, and rituals . . . to predict risks and communicate knowledge about avoiding hazards," the modern field of risk studies

and communication "developed from the practical needs of indus-
trialized societies to regulate technology and to protect its citizens
from natural and manmade, technological hazards" (Palenchar, 2009,
p. 32). With governmental campaigns of the 1950s, such as "Atoms for
Peace" (p. 32), and the passing of the Federal Disaster Relief Act of
1950 (Henkey, 2017, p. 18), the United States entered into a more systematized period of risk assessment and response that included a more
formalized organizational structure responsible for federal response
to broadly conceived emergencies; however, the history of emergency
preparedness at the national level is one that is mired in overlapping
departments working at cross-purposes (p. 19). Even after passing the
1974 Disaster Relief Act, "multiple federal agencies [were] in charge of
vaguely defined portions of disaster planning, response, and recovery"
(p. 19). In 1978, it was proposed that a number of federal departments
and agencies merge to create the Federal Emergency Management
Agency (FEMA); this became finalized in 1979, less than a week after
the Three Mile Island incident (p. 20–21). The 1980s, then, became
a watershed moment for both risk communication and emergency
response in which federal power over disaster and emergency declara-
tions, eligibility criteria, and emergency assistance to state and local
governments was consolidated to the executive branch through autho-
rization of the Stafford Act (1988) (p. 22). The 1990s saw the Clinton
administration appoint the first emergency management professional
to run FEMA. During this period, FEMA focused heavily on "mitigation, preparedness, and response/recovery" (p. 23).

   The historical discombobulation of American emergency planning
has contributed to ongoing and current issues plaguing emergency
planning and response teams. One such issue is the lack of coordinated
planning and response to emergencies from the municipal and state
levels up to federal ones (think here about the lack of coordinated
emergency response between local, state, and federal agencies during
the 9/11 attacks, Hurricane Katrina, and the Virginia Tech shooting).
Another issue is the mission of federal emergency planning shut-
tling between military and civic focuses. Post-9/11, the Department of
Homeland Security was established, with FEMA rolled into this mainly
terrorism-focused super-agency (p. 24). Around this time, mitigation
and preparedness took a backseat to response and recovery at the
agency (p. 25). So, yet another issue is FEMA's reactive rather than proactive approach to emergency planning and response; this less effective
reactive approach has made its way into other sectors that engage in
emergency planning, such as higher education.

EMERGENCY PLANNING IN AMERICAN HIGHER EDUCATION

Colleges and universities began engaging in systematized risk assessment, emergency planning, and communication in formalized ways around the beginning of the 21st century. However, as Bruxvoort (2012) notes, a 2006 survey found that higher-education institutions had major gaps in their emergency preparedness, including that most institutions were only prepared for emergencies they had experienced before (p. 100). While institutions learned from past experiences, they struggled to "apply that experience in a broader context" (p. 100). Crisis management, at this time, was relatively undersupported compared with other institutional programs (p. 100).

Since the mid-aughts, the field of emergency preparedness has made inroads in high education insofar as it has become a more established and routine part of its organizational structure and work. Scholars cite profound tragedies that spurred the development of institutional and governmental policies around emergency response, such as the rape and murder of Jeanne Cleary in 1986, which led to the Cleary Act (1998), and the Virginia Tech massacre (2007), which led to an amendment of the Cleary Act (2008) to require the development and implementation of emergency response plans across higher education, as well as the development of emergency alert systems to coordinate emergency response with community members (Kapucu & Khosa, 2013, p. 2).

It is really only in the last decade or so that emergency response has become formalized in higher education. This is because visible and wide-ranging emergencies on college campuses have contributed to a demand for coordinated planning and response; it is also because, as Sattler et al. (2014) suggest, "emergency incidents are becoming more frequent on college campuses and place students, faculty, and staff in harm's way" (p. 258). Recent research on university and college emergency planning and response have found that "80 percent now have some sort of threat assessment team, more than 90 per cent have emergency response plans in place, and many have lockdown plans" (Regehr et al., 2017, p. 75). My own experience in higher education tracks with these findings insofar as all the colleges and universities where I have worked over the last 12 years or so have had structures in place to assess risks and plan for emergencies, including emergency planning committees, working groups, programs, and even departments; however, prior to this point, when I was a student, emergency plans were either completely absent from my college experience, or they were not widely disseminated. A lot has changed, then, in a relatively short amount of time in terms of how colleges and universities assess, plan, and address

Table 5.1. The Ohio State University's list of top 10 hazard risks in order of likelihood of occurrence in and around Columbus, Ohio

1	Fire
2	Severe Thunderstorm/Tornado
3	Cyber Attack
4	Electrical Failure
5	Bomb/Violence Threat
6	Snowfall
7	Active Shooter
8	Ice Storm
9	Flooding
10	Civil Unrest

emergencies, due to legislative action as well as cultural shifts around the culture of risk and hazard on college campuses.

But even when plans are in place for specific emergencies, as Bruxvoort (2012) notes, there can be many gaps regarding events that have never occurred before at a school. As Fifolt et al. (2016) suggest, "emergency management for U.S. higher education institutions is complex because the range of potential hazards and disasters is almost limitless" and requires an "all-hazards" approach to emergency management that is similar to governmental agencies (p. 61). For example, a recent report (2017) from Ohio State that includes a hazard vulnerability analysis (Table 5.1) developed their rankings by considering "probability and severity of a given hazard" (p. 5). A variety of information goes into risk assessment such as geographic, political, actuarial, and other data to identify the likely occurrence of emergencies. Among the top 10 hazards, active shooters are not ranked as highly as more mundane but equally dangerous events such as weather-related risks. And knife attacks are not included at all. Similarly, pandemics do not make it to the list of top 10 potential hazards, even though we are currently facing a worldwide pandemic (COVID-19) which is unprecedented in our lifetime.

Thus, preparation for emergencies includes anticipating a wide variety of risks (all-hazards), some of which are not caused by humans but are nevertheless dangerous to us. Furthermore, risk assessment can be informed by highly localized data, such as past hazardous events, current geopolitical climate, current geophysical climate, and so on. But it should also be informed by expansive consideration of potential and hitherto unseen risks and emergencies. In developing an emergency plan, consider the kinds of risks in the environment and how likely they are to occur at the micro level as well as the macro level. As I suggest elsewhere, writing centers are unique both in spatial arrangement and in their utilization by workers and clients; therefore, localized risk at the site might differ from the broader institutional risks. Considering different levels of risk potentiality, then, makes sense when developing a departmental emergency plan. What might a survey of your writing center's hazards ranking that assesses both "probability and severity of a given hazard" (p. 5) yield?

PLANNING BEFORE, DURING, AND AFTER EMERGENCIES

Given that the field of emergency planning is relatively young in higher education and, also, that many emergency plans do not account for the micro level in their guidance, I provide an outlined template for developing an emergency plan (Appendix D). Information for this plan was developed in concert with a number of emergency plans and suggested templates, including from FEMA, Ohio State, and Nova Scotia Department of Education.

I also include elements in the emergency plan template that come from my research on wellness and care in writing center work. After my experience with the active aggressor situation, I came to several conclusions about emergency planning. For one, there are notable absences in OSU's departmental plans regarding post-emergency response. My staff and I were hungry to process our experiences of crisis and to reevaluate how we respond in emergencies even though there were no protocols in official documents provided by the university to do so, and we ultimately processed in an ad hoc way that semester; therefore, I added a "Post-Emergency: Wellbeing and Recovery" section to my emergency plan template that is largely derived from the experience of feeling rudderless in the aftermath of a traumatic and broadly affecting event. Included in this plan are mindfulness and contemplative practice training, which we learned about in our staff workshops during the 2017–2018 academic year, and which helped us to process our experiences with the active aggressor situation. Similarly, I added a necessary section to pre-semester orientation on protocols for calling campus security and police ("Planning Before an Emergency"), because protocols on how to engage with law enforcement—especially when there are staff and clients of color present—were absent from emergency plans although there was implicit involvement by police and other law enforcement in managing crises, which was made apparent in many of the emergency plans I reviewed.

Therefore, the emergency plan resource I provide includes the more typical things that one would expect in such a guide alongside those that are informed by my research, as well as by my tutors, who pushed me to think through implications of relying on police and campus security in times of crisis for staff and students of color. Below, I identify some of the elements of this emergency planning guide and offer contextualization for why inclusion of these topics is pivotal in planning, managing, and processing crises.

INTRODUCTION TO EMERGENCY PLAN/PLANNING

Most people do not have training in risk assessment and emergency planning; therefore, it is critical that any development of a plan begins with stakeholder conversations that give the context for developing such a plan, define characteristics of an emergency, anticipate some potential risks, and clearly articulate the plan's goals and uses. In order to get people to participate in emergency planning, and increase responsiveness and decrease conflicts within an organization,

> risk communication should not be seen as a top-down activity in which experts educate the public about risks but rather as an interactive process characterized by a multi-factor flow of information on risks and the meaning each actor attributes to the risks. (Gutteling, 2000, p. 240)

Of course, the director/administrator can brainstorm different elements or key information that ought to go into such a plan, but it is critical to set the expectation that this is a "living document" that is continuously reviewed, revised, discussed, and shared among center stakeholders.

I also share a caveat here that a lot of schools already have campus-wide emergency plans, and some might have zoned plans or building-level plans. As with my experience, however, these plans might not be widely shared, easily accessed, or pertinent to specific organization sites (such as a writing center and its various locations). Therefore, when developing a center plan, it is also critical to consult any emergency planning boards, committees, or taskforces and to have discussions with other community members who are responsible for developing and carrying out these emergency plans. All of this upfront work is time consuming, but it is critical that any emergency plan is vetted by campus-wide administration. In fact, I would make the argument, if it is not already expected, that individual units should have a heavy hand in developing their own emergency plans, especially since the physical spaces on campus vary widely, as do the kinds of people who occupy those spaces.

Writing centers are incredibly idiosyncratic spaces with very high levels of use including long-term use (tutoring sessions) as well as short-term use (foot traffic between sessions and tutor shifts, etc.). They also have widely varying kinds of spatial layouts and configurations and can be co-located in other public spaces and/or distributed across campus. Our writing center, for example, had three physical locations, one that was open-concept (tutors occupied tables in the library during drop-in hours), one that was a converted physics lab with multiple small rooms that lacked dividers (but included four or so doors that were routinely locked and that opened out onto a hallway), and one that was open-concept but shared space in a veterans' lounge (with glass windows and doors and no secondary exit). In each of these sites, different safety protocols needed to be developed in concert with other departments and units on campus, such as Military and Veterans Services and libraries. As we see with the history of emergency response at the federal level, as well as some key breakdowns during crisis management, such as at Virginia Tech, the hierarchical and individualistic nature of emergency planning and response can adversely affect crisis response; therefore, it is critical to communicate across departments and share one's emergency planning documents widely among all kinds of stakeholders that are internal and external to the writing center.

It is also critical, because staff can be distributed across many different localities, to include wayfinding details for each site in emergency planning and other center-wide documents. At OSU, tutors did site walk-throughs before the start of the semester and identified how to access exits, fire extinguishers, first aid kits, elevators, the basement level, and pertinent administrative documents, such as staff contact lists, safety documentation, and support documents (such as OSU's "Guide to Assist Distressed Individuals"). We also included visual and textual maps of our locations on our website for both tutors and clients to access. Some of these wayfinding resources serve multiple purposes; in addition to assisting with emergency planning, for staff, they also give clients and tutors a sense of the accessibility level for each writing center location.

Emergency Plans Tend to Include the Following:
- Emergency coordinator (main contact)
- Emergency communications systems for staff (e.g., email, phone tree, Slack, etc.)
- Emergency preparedness information
- Spatial information (exits, basement access, first aid kit locations, fire extinguisher location, etc.)
- Evacuation plan (which includes plans for supporting persons with disabilities)
- Protocols for specific emergencies such as:
  - How to evacuate the building due to a gas leak
  - How to evacuative the building due to a fire
  - How to shelter in place during a tornado warning
  - How to respond during an active shooter event

It is Critical to:

- Involve internal and external stakeholders in plan development
- Share the plan with all staff
- Discuss the plan
- Regularly review and update the plan
- Know and follow shelter-in-place guidelines (and other policies) of your institution
- Account for long-term crises in emergency planning
- Develop post-emergency procedures and resources such as counseling, leave time, and contemplative practices

PLANNING BEFORE AN EMERGENCY

Define Emergency Terms for Staff

After the active aggressor situation, it came out that there was widespread confusion regarding the definition of "run, hide, fight." Community members said they were confused about when to engage in which action. Similarly, during the emergency, news outlets were suggesting barricading doors, even though this is a tactic used in the fight stage rather than in the run or even hide stages of an active aggressor situation. For example, the Writing Center at OSU has multiple doors—many of which are not regularly used and which open to a hallway. However, barricading the wrong door might have made egress impossible. So, before an emergency strikes, it is critical to have a plan and discuss that plan—including explaining emergency planning concepts and defining them—as during a crisis, pressure might come from family, friends, and media outlets hundreds or thousands of miles away to act in ways that are counter to on-the-ground advice. Following the guidelines put out by the institution is paramount.

Explaining Emergency Notification Systems

It is essential to have quick access to the contact information of every employee at the WC, which includes both an email list—to communicate out quickly, advising those not yet on campus to stay away until they are given the official "all clear"—but also to have access to staff phone numbers in order to contact those who might already be on campus but not in a protected space. Emailing out to staff helped ensure that those who were not on campus did not unintentionally walk into an active emergency. During the Virginia Tech shooting in 2007, students were not warned and came onto campus and were murdered. Emergency notification systems became standard for higher education following that event. However, large schools like OSU often send out batched alerts; therefore, even if your school has an emergency notification system, it is important to communicate expectations (particularly that safety supersedes work obligations) to writing center tutors. This is especially important if a writing center has many tutors that are also international students. At OSU, tutors from other countries were far more concerned with missing their shifts than they were with the lockdown and shelter-in-place orders. Cultural and societal differences among staff make it critical that expectations for behavior during an emergency are clearly communicated and that all tutors are contacted as a secondary precaution, in addition to pre-emergency training. And, of course, if your school does not have an emergency notification system, immediately advocate for your institution to set one up.

Clarify Emergency Planning Training Resources and Expectations

There are many institution-specific training initiatives on emergency preparedness. At OSU, we required every tutor to do the following:

- Review the active shooter video.
- Review the guide to assisting distressed individuals.
- Engage in Title IX training.
- Engage in suicide prevention training.
- Engage in recognizing students struggling with crisis training.
- For those working with veterans, we asked them to take an online training on this population and their unique experiences and needs.

In addition to these trainings, I also created a workshop on emergency planning that included discussion scenarios (Appendix E) that were based on real events that were specific to our writing center. I also developed a workshop that addressed how tutors should respond in specific crises that was based on Ohio State Department of Public Safety's Emergency Procedures Guide. While some of these trainings were institutionally sponsored, some were specific to the Writing Center. It is critical, as my research on wellness training has found, to engage a variety of training and resource guides and that some, if not all, of these are contextualized for the uniqueness of writing center work. Training tutors using emergency preparedness or Title IX resources that are crafted for students leaves out critical information for how student workers respond to crises. For example, all employees at OSU, including student workers, are mandatory reporters of Title IX violations; therefore, the unique position that student workers occupy demands novel training and resources that acknowledge and account for their liminal position on campus and that articulates their workplace responsibilities alongside their responsibilities as students.

Ramifications of Involvement of Police/Campus Security in Emergencies

Responding to emergencies by calling campus security and/or the police has often been an action recommended by writing centers that I have worked in and, despite my own reluctance to call the police because of personal experiences growing up in New York City, I also advocated for this action with tutors at my first job, if they faced dangerous situations. However, as countless scholars and news media outlets have reported, the act of calling the police can have deadly consequences for people of color who are in proximity to the area, or, in the case of "racially motivated police reporting" (McNamarah, 2019, p. 335). Recent Black Lives Matter protests, as well as protests from the inception of the movement in the mid-2010s, protest the police murdering Black people for simply existing (walking, running, sleeping, sitting in their yard). To prevent further victims of what McNamarah calls "white caller crime" reporting (p. 335), we need to develop clear policies around calling the police/campus security to the writing center.

Tutors of color brought this matter to me during our development of emergency planning trainings and while we did not issue a blanket statement against calling the police during emergencies, we did set up clear protocols for doing so that would minimize harm to our tutors and clients of color. First, we discussed the ramifications of calling campus security (who carry firearms at OSU) for different groups of people who work and utilize the Writing Center. Then, we determined under what specific circumstances one might call. Finally, we determined that a community care approach to this decision would be one to adopt. Tutors and center leaders who felt empowered to call the police and/or who were not afraid or distrustful of the police agreed to step up and call in the event of an emergency but only after announcing their intentions to call the police to other center occupants (tutors and clients). This way, tutors and clients of color had the option of leaving the space prior to the arrival of security. The discussion around determining if and when campus security is needed in the Writing Center allowed us to have a discussion about our community's stance on policing and empowered tutors of color to voice their concerns with defaulting to them in times of emergencies. While arguments for defunding the police and removing campus security (and their weapons) altogether from college campuses have become more popularized, this was not the discussion taking place at our institution at the time. At the time, we navigated some of the challenges of living in a Republican-controlled state with permissive gun laws (campus security carried guns on campus) by developing an emergency plan that accounted for tutors and clients of color, particularly Black tutors and clients, which was critical work. So, in any emergency plan, it is critical that WCAs work to include marginalized people such as people of color, queer and trans people, and people with disabilities, as these are the groups that often face additional dangers during emergencies (and, well, in daily life).

As a note, when I arrived at Middlebury College, I again tried to have a conversation about campus policing in the hope that we could set a similar or even more radical policy about the role of policing during emergencies. However, during our emergency planning discussion, my undergraduate tutors (who, at the time, were majority white and largely upper-middle to upper class) were reluctant to discuss policing and insisted that they had never had issues with campus police. Since the murder of George Floyd, of course, there have been student-led petitions and committees dedicated to abolishing police on campus. So, I see this issue as one that is ongoing and that tutors might not be comfortable addressing in public spaces. Therefore, one way to develop an inclusive emergency plan is to create an anonymous survey that allows tutors to identify the different kinds of things they are concerned about both during emergencies but also in their everyday lived experiences on campus and in the writing center. Just because an issue is not openly discussed does not mean that it isn't roiling under the surface or that conversations are not taking place elsewhere on campus. To create policies around policing on campus, have individual discussions with tutors, connect with groups like Black Student Union, Queer Alliance, and other groups dedicated to this work, and, again, do the hard work of talking about this topic regularly over time.

Employee Expectations and Responsibilities During an Emergency

After the active aggressor situation, I realized we had few clear procedures for how to respond in emergencies. There was little to no guidance on navigating our spaces, determining evacuation protocols, or how to aid people with disabilities in the event of evacuation. Also, the duties of staff—especially student workers—during emergencies were unclear. Because of all these uncertainties, I developed a set of trainings that I mention earlier in this chapter. In addition to developing discussion scenarios for tutors to work through how they would respond to complex and realistic emergencies (Appendix E), I created a workshop on emergency planning. I also met with campus security and discussed the roles that employees have in large-scale emergencies. Similar to FEMA and other risk-minded governmental institutions, employees are the first line of defense in local emergencies. Even OSU's website on emergency planning (2019) recognizes that staff are likely to be on the front lines during crises, as they note on the website, "You are the first line of defense, the eyes and ears watching out for the safety of Ohio State. All of us must take responsibility for our own safety and assist those around us" (The Ohio State University, 2019). In other words, in an emergency, community members and volunteers are typically the first to respond, sometimes well in advance of government or other official agencies (p. 1–2), especially if the emergency is one that precludes top-down support from arriving in a timely manner.

The training I developed refers heavily to local, state, and university emergency planning guidelines and resources. While state and local municipalities tend to have legal mutual aid agreements allowing them to collaborate on emergency response, "colleges and universities are generally excluded from these laws due to their status as either private or state-supported institutions rather than local governmental entities" (Schloss & Cragg, 2013, p. 255); therefore, responses to emergencies might differ from entity to entity (e.g., university-, municipal-, and state-level agencies) and there might be little coordination between response efforts. It's important, then, to plug into different emergency-response systems and to identify which response team to follow during an emergency. Of course, lines of reportage and communication should be determined prior to when an emergency occurs.

To bring these discussions down to the micro level of the writing center, I developed scenarios for discussion (Appendix E) that were taken from real-life emergencies that occurred at OSU, which helped tutors to contextulize emergencies within the scope of their everyday lived experiences. Additionally, I developed a set of questions that helped tutors think about the spaces they work in every day from the standpoint of emergency planning and risk assessment. These included noticing the location of key and potentially lifesaving things such as fire alarms, fire extinguishers, exits, basements, and first aid kits and think about under what circumstances to utilize these things.

Here Are Some Prompts on Spatial Awareness and Emergency Planning:
- Where is the nearest fire alarm?
- Where is the nearest fire extinguisher?
- Where is the first aid kid?
- Where is the nearest exit, and what would be your exit route?
- How would you shelter in place in this room (the Writing Center)?
- What would you do during the following emergencies:
  - Tornado warning
  - Chemical or biological agent
  - Active shooter alert

While conversations on these topics might seem stressful—WCAs might worry that they are placing undue burdens on their tutors—I have found that undergraduate and graduate tutors display great maturity in talking about emergency planning, perhaps more so than discussing topics such as mental health concerns, stress, and other wellness-related topics. While I have little empirical research on why this may be, I imagine it is because tutors are often quite altruistic and community-oriented (and data from the wellness study does show tutors' positive feelings toward writing center work and toward their colleagues); therefore, they do well with reasoning through emergency scenarios and considering the roles they would take during crises, because these impact their colleagues and their clients in addition to themselves.

EMERGENCY RESPONSE EXPECTATIONS FOR PEER TUTORS

Of course, designating responsibility in an emergency is complicated—do you designate team leaders who handle crises as they arise? Do you discuss blanket expectations for all tutors regarding how they handle emergencies? Do you take on the responsibility entirely, as a director or administrator? I provide training that offers standard behavioral practices for all tutors but then offer one-on-one discussions and group meetings for center leadership (graduate and undergraduate assistant directors) that include additional responsibilities. Of course, any responsibilities that are designated to center workers should be in compliance with institution-wide rules. And, when in doubt, consult with these stakeholders before assigning duties.

Evacuation

I advise tutors that, in the case of punctuated and short-term emergencies, they should evacuate and seek safety. For example, when we had a gas leak in the center, tutors took their belongings and proceeded to the exits. They did not return to the building to complete their shifts, instead canceling their appointments. One tutor moved their session to the library, which did not have a gas leak, but this was above and beyond expectations. Most emergencies require following sensible and prede-termined actions, many of which involve getting to safety. To this end, whenever possible, I have encouraged tutors to evacuate to seek safety during emergencies. In addition to identifying scenarios in which it is appropriate to evacuate (fire, gas leak, bomb threat, etc.), we identify evacuation routes, meet-up locations (and when meeting is necessary), and how to evacuate persons with disabilities. However, in the event that evacuation is not possible, we discuss other precautions and actions one can take in response to an emergency, such as during a nearby active aggressor situation (run, hide), or a tornado warning (sheltering in place on the lower levels of buildings), and so on.

On the Importance of Saying "No" in a Crisis

During certain crises, saying "no" is critical. During the active aggres-sor situation, there were clients and consultants who just wanted to leave, but we were 0.2 miles from the active area and most of the roads around our building were closed. There were snipers on the roofs and helicopters circling overhead. And, as much as I also wanted to get out of the Writing Center, I followed what I believed to be the lockdown guidelines for the school and had to simply say "no"—no to leaving, no to drawing attention to our space, no to requests for the bathroom and water fountains and all the other comforts we are used to. Panic often makes people want to act with impulse rather than forethought. To com-bat panic in the center, I asked a tutor and a client to hold a session in my office (lights out, shades drawn, of course). I listened to the police scanner and to local and national media outlets and reported updates to other tutors and clients. I even poured juice and soda for everyone to try to keep them a little bit more comfortable. Once we were given the all-clear, I asked everyone to develop a personal evacuation plan (buses, cars, and other vehicles weren't allowed on campus) and communicate it with me. We then vacated the building in small groups.

I did not take these actions to normalize the situation we were in but instead to calm any feelings of panic and to avoid any impulsive and reactive behavior. I also, as noted above, said "no" to a number of requests for tutors and clients to leave the center. After the event, I found out that educators cannot require adults (those over 18 years old) to comply with shelter-in-place orders. This poses very real dangers for those in compliance with shelter-in-place orders during active aggressor situations, particularly when following the "hide" protocol. I cannot purport to have the right answers for addressing this complexity; it is a matter of instinct versus legality. My suggestion here is to consult with various external stakeholders to understand just what kind of authority and responsibilities you have during crises. I am sure they vary from one institution to another.

POST-EMERGENCY: WELLBEING AND RECOVERY

An under-focused-on area of emergency planning is what to do once the crisis has abated. Of course, with COVID-19, we are also seeing a lack of preparation for handling long-term crises that do not really "go away" but linger over very long periods of time. However, we know that one's experience of an emergency in the moment might be quite different from one's experience after the emergency has ended or, in the case of long-term emergencies, over the course of time. Therefore, it is critical to include appreciable guidance and plans for post-emergency response. Some ideas for how to do this work might include offering listening sessions in which community members get together and reflect on the crisis and how it was managed. This, of course, might lead to refinement of the emergency plan. However, it is also important to have discussions that simply make space for the feelings that come along with crisis.

At OSU, it seemed, there were always crises. After the active aggressor situation, gun-rights advocates marched on the Oval with semiautomatic weapons. Then, there were multiple rounds of white supremacist fliers posted around campus with individual people targeted. There were, while I was there, at least seven suicides and at least three students murdered. We also had multiple tornado warnings, an arctic blast that shut down school, and a snowstorm or two that should have shut it down. I list these things because there are many different types of emergencies. There are the widespread emergencies, and then there are personal emergencies, such as tutors who experience the death of a family member, or who struggle with coming out, or who experience sexual assault. As we know from Degner et al.'s (2015) work on mental health concerns, tutors carry their experiences with them into the center and into their work. Therefore, reflective work post-emergency allows for a kind of check-in that can help WCAs determine if tutors need support, flex time, or a community to lean on.

Some Ideas for Post-Emergency Well-being Work Includes:

- Town hall–style meeting about the handling of the emergency (might lead to revision of plan)
- Small-group discussions
- Individual one-on-one discussions
- Reflective group activity (free writing, creative writing, bullet journaling)
- Contemplative activities (yoga session, meditation session, breathing session) lead by trained professionals
- Creation of case studies/after-action reports that utilize storytelling

CONCLUSION

Writing can be used in a wide variety of ways to respond to crisis. More specifically, scholars have explored the role of storytelling in emergency management education (Jerolleman, 2020). Storytelling, as we see with Our Marathon, the Boston Marathon bombing public archive, can be used to report out after an emergency, but it can also be used to memorialize, to plan, to educate, to reflect, and to community-build. Consider how the writing center can support its members in processing their experiences of the emergency and, also, how these documents can serve educational purposes for future tutors. One regret I have is that I had so many one-on-one conversations after the various emergencies our center experienced rather than getting the entire group together for a larger discussion and reflection section. In subsequent years of emergency planning training, tutors were able to offer their experiences but, due to worker turnover, these experiences were often individualistic rather than communal.

I often felt responsible, because of my unique position as director, for the continuity portion of crisis management, which is draining work. While some among us might believe that emergency planning and risk assessment is not the work of educators, as I have noted throughout this book, the neoliberal institution demands its workers to be agile and to move quickly—and often with little preparation—into new roles. While I do not believe that the writing administrator should be the *only* source of support during emergencies, my personal experience as well as my research on the structures of emergency response teams at the institutional and government levels have taught me that in times of crisis there might not be other people around to help us. So, while my inclination might be to buck job duty creep, I also recognize that emergencies are the norm—not the exception—in our world. My hope is that this chapter will help us to develop nuanced and thoughtful emergency plans that prepare for a range of potential emergencies but that also allow us to process trauma and other experiences, post-crisis. Planning for emergencies—and recognizing how one's subjectivity and lived experiences affect our responses to crisis—will, I hope, help us to treat ourselves with kindness and care when the next crisis comes around.

PART III

Looking to the Future of Wellness Work

6

TOWARD AN INTERSECTIONAL PRAXIS OF EMOTIONAL LABOR IN WRITING CENTERS

OPENING NARRATIVE

The work we do can deplete us even if we are not currently struggling with large-scale crises. The ways in which we currently work in our society, which are impacted by neoliberalism but also by disaster capitalism and constructed precarity, all affect how we engage with work. Yet many of us are just grateful to get a job in academia once completing our degree work. So, while a lot of this book has discussed the ways in which external factors are brought to bear on our everyday lived work experiences, internal factors such as one's childhood, one's work experiences, and one's class background also affect our experience of work in the present moment.

Before I became interested in wellness, I did not think much about how emotions figure into my work. Being from a working-class family, I was raised with the expectation that work was a point of pride in one's life but, then again, it also produced suffering, which my family also framed as a point of pride. There was little discussion of work as pleasurable or intellectually fulfilling. Despite moving away from blue collar work to do academic work, I have, for most of my professional life, carried around these assumptions about how individuals relate to their jobs. I have thrown myself headlong into work without thinking too deeply about how I perform it. I have felt a sense of pride at over-extending myself or otherwise going above and beyond job expectations. It is only recently that I have been thinking about the ramifications of drawing upon and depleting my emotional and physical resources to shore up and perform my job duties.

At the beginning of this book, I talked about how many WCAs—and educators, broadly speaking—are not trained to handle the mess of wellness needs that arise in their daily working lives. Here, I also acknowledge that academics are not really trained to distinguish between their

https://doi.org/10.7330/9781646423606.c006

labor and their "love" (emotionality). A lot of times, these are presented to us during our professionalization period as one and the same. I took this labor of love rhetoric to heart. When it was still theoretical, I spoke often with my partner about having to "go wherever the job is," yet when the time came, I desperately tried to stay in New England—the region where I spent my emergent adulthood. Labor and love, I realized, need to be separated, as they are not one and the same.

In my first job, at a community college, I heavily relied upon my subjectivity and emotionality to do my job. A first-generation college graduate who had taken community college classes, I believed that I could only mentor and support my students and my tutors through sharing my stories and mentoring them through empathy. At the same time, I confronted a lot of what I now recognize as burnout rhetoric coming from some of my more frustrated colleagues when they emailed or stopped me in the hallway to complain about one of their students' inability to write. I share this rather mundane example about how writing centers are perceived by some faculty as opposed to the lifeline they can be for tutors and students (and, even, some WCAs, faculty, staff, etc.) because of how common these kinds of interactions are for WCAs. Carter (2009) shares a similar story to detail how common complaints about literacy instruction are political as much as they are pedagogical in nature (p. 135). After every experience where writing center work was devalued, a part of me that overly identified with the students and the center was hurt. I cannot say that I have been entirely able to divorce myself from feeling profound pain (and a healthy dose of anger) in response to these kinds of aggressions but, lately, I am far less likely than I once was to think I am doing something wrong when a faculty member complains about a student, a tutor, or the Writing Center. Recognizing how my emotions figure into my labor—and separating my self-concept from my work—has allowed me to develop critical distance between these things.

In this chapter, I share scholarship on the roots of emotional labor and frame how writing centers—by virtue of their organizational structures, their mission, their training, and their services—can be identified as workplaces that require emotional labor from their staff. I also talk about how Hochschild's research into emotional labor is underpinned by class-based socialization including specific norms and expectations around managing one's emotions. That these patterns are often rooted in one's formative experiences and home life has deep implications for how writing centers both recruit and support people from working-class backgrounds alongside those from middle- and upper-class backgrounds. Finally, as I mention in my narrative, I further detail how to identify and manage workplace burnout—something I was not attuned to as a new faculty member but have become well-acquainted with over the past years.

LITERATURE REVIEW
Emotional Labor and Burnout

Emotional labor is a phrase that was coined by sociologist Arlie Hochschild in her book *The Managed Heart* (2012). Originally published in 1983, Hochschild defined emotional labor as the kind of work that is bound up with "the *emotional style of offering the service*" (p. 19). Emotional labor, then, is the additional affective work that employers expect their employees to perform to do their job satisfactorily; "Seeming to 'love the job' becomes part of the job" (p. 19). Hochschild identifies three criteria for classifying emotional labor in particular jobs:

> First, they require face-to-face or voice-to-voice contact with the public. Second, they require the worker to produce an emotional state in another person—gratitude or fear, for example. Third, they allow the employer, through training and supervision, to exercise a degree of control over the emotional activities of employees. (p. 102)

There is variation in how jobs are classified as requiring emotional labor, with specific workers within these jobs engaging in more or less of this kind of work.

Before the publication of *The Managed Heart* (2012), Hochschild wrote, "Emotion work, feeling rules, and social structure" (1979), which argues that emotional regulation is profoundly influenced by class and other social structures, which, in turn, prepare us for specific kinds of jobs that require more or less emotional regulation; therefore, "social exchange, commoditization of feeling, and the premium, in many middle-class jobs, on the capacity to manage meanings" (p. 569) gives rise to a recapitulation of class structures in how we emote, the kinds of jobs we secure, how we work, and how we emote while we work.

This "occupational demand on feeling" (1979, p. 25) that Hochschild describes, is part of "the toe and the heel of capitalism," which is a metaphor that explains the dynamic present in corporations and other kinds of business (p. 25). The toe delivers the service, and the heel collects payment for it (p. 96). What Hochschild identifies, then, is how class affects peoples' abilities to emotionally regulate, and, in turn, this drives people to jobs that are either more "toe"-oriented or more "heel"-oriented. Emotional labor is required of many public-facing jobs, as her criteria suggests; however, it is especially an expected element of many middle-class white-collar jobs. Writing centers fall under the "toe" dynamic in which a service is delivered, often with kindness; though one might see the larger systemic forces that produced modern writing centers (Boquet, 1999), and that drive many students to the writing center, through disciplinary action, such as faculty requirements, university expectations, and inflexible literacy standards, as a kind of "heel" that collects upon the (emotional) labor of the writing center.

Since Hochschild, emotional labor has been studied in several different spaces. The term has been used incorrectly (Beck, 2018; West, 2019) to describe invisible and unpaid labor that is performed by women and other marginalized groups. It has been studied in professional fields traditionally identified as "helping professions" (Graf et al., 2014) or jobs whose main goal it is to "nurture the growth of, or address the problems of a persons [*sic*] physical, psychological, intellectual or emotional constitution" (p. 2), including teaching (Lee, 2019; Lindqvist et al., 2019; Zaretsky & Katz, 2019), medicine (Vinson & Underman, 2020), and mental health (Hings et al., 2020), among others. As the interest in emotional labor has increased in other helping professions, including a number related to education work, it has also been addressed in writing center studies.

While the recent COVID-19 crisis has given rise to a number of conversations about labor taking place on social media, on listservs, and in virtual meet-ups—including about emotional labor, invisible labor, compensated labor, and unethical labor—there is also a growing body of scholarly research on this topic in writing center studies. One seminal study, Caswell et al.'s (2016) *The Working Lives of New Writing Center Directors*, engages in a case study approach to interviewing new writing center directors in order to trace how "participants experienced their jobs in terms of emotion" (p. 10). The authors found that "the case studies revealed facets of writing center director labor that other types of research or scholarship have up to now left invisible" (p. 10). Another is the edited collection on emotional labor in writing program administration, *The Things We Carry: Strategies for Recognizing and Negotiating Emotional Labor in Writing Program Administration* (Wooten et al., 2020), which offers a set of strategy sheets for managing emotional labor, engaging in ethical WPA work, and responding to crises and disasters.

Around 2015, however, other scholars were also writing about the different ways in which writing center workers—particularly tutors—experience and engage in emotional labor. Nicklay (2012) studies tutors' guilt when they act counter to perceived writing center orthodoxies, such as engaging in directive tutoring approaches. Perry (2016) recognizes how writing center administrators grapple with emotional labor as a facet of their job but also as a facet of tutors' work:

> As directors, we are aware that, while we can never entirely alleviate or compensate the real emotional labor involved in the job of talking with students one-on-one about the often-vexing subject of their writing, there are some things we can do to support and care for our staff as they go about their work. (p. 2)

Similarly, Rowell (2015) wrote a thesis entitled *Let's Talk Emotions: Re-Envisioning the Writing Center Through Consultant Emotional Labor*, which found that "consultants often engage in emotional labor through expressing positive emotions and suppressing negative emotions by using a variety of emotional management strategies" (p. 1). In 2018, Neisha-Anne Green published a piece on the unique experiences of writing center workers of color and the emotional toll of navigating predominately white and white-supremacist spaces as a Black person. Green's piece is one of the first to explicitly address issues of emotional labor and burnout from the perspective of a Black person who engages in writing center work. Since then, WLN published a special issue on wellness that addressed issues of emotional labor and attendant emotional management, such as tutors-in-training experiencing work-related anxiety (Emmelhainz, 2020), administrators avoiding burnout while managing mentor relationships (Concannon et al., 2020), and tutors setting boundaries to avoid additional emotional labor (Parsons, 2020).

EXAMINING EMOTIONAL LABOR IN WRITING CENTERS

As this body of research demonstrates, there are a lot of feelings in and around writing centers that are related to how tutors and administrators experience their work; therefore, it is necessary to parse the kinds of feelings that occur in writing centers and compare them with Hochschild's (1979) criteria for identifying emotional labor. As she notes, jobs that require emotional labor:

- Are often public-facing
- "Allow the employer, through training and supervision, to exercise a degree of control over the emotional activities of employees" (p. 102)
- Require the "worker to produce an emotional state in another person" (p. 102)

Writing centers require an immense amount of one-on-one engagement with people (in higher education or otherwise). In fact, the basis of tutoring work is rooted in individual consultations or sessions. And, often, even if our centers do not work with the general public outside the institution, we still field queries and needs from them. Requests for editors, questions about grammar, demands for tutoring sessions, and other kinds of needs come across the desks of many writing centers regularly. In fact, in every writing center that I have worked, I have fielded countless requests from the public for support and access to services far outside the scope of what the writing center could provide. So, even in spaces where interfacing with the public—outside of the university community—is not necessarily a main mission of a writing center, our services are often one of the first points of contact for community needs related to literacy and other support.

Writing center tutors are often trained to manage the expectations and needs of clients, which includes training on learning how to say "no" to unrealistic or unethical demands (Parsons, 2020), learning how to manage emotionally charged sessions such as when clients cry (Gillespie & Lerner, 2008, p. 177), and learning how to manage other "what if?" scenarios that may occur when writing center work does not go smoothly (Gillespie & Lerner, 2008). Additionally, as much of the wellness training that I have designed for my centers demonstrates, training might also include a host of other ways to manage tutors' affective responses to specific tutoring situations, particularly in instances where clients are disruptive or distressed. However, even at a basic organizational level, many writing centers rely upon a public-facing and in-person model that often includes intake approaches modeled on customer service—or the therapeutic intake model. Therefore, even when we might not realize we are doing it, we are often training and supervising our tutors' emotional activities and asking them to respond in specific ways to crises, emergencies, or other affective moments that arise in the center.

The final criterion for identifying emotional labor is the requirement that the worker must "produce an emotional state in another person" (Hochschild, 1979, p. 102). Returning to the toe and heel analogy, I have often felt like writing centers, with their ethos of care, frame their work within an affective model. This places pressure upon writing center workers—especially tutors, but also WCAs—to elicit specific kinds of positive feelings in and around the writing center. However, overlaid onto their pressure to perform positive or good feelings toward the writing center, and in return to receive such feedback from clients, there is also the pressure that tutors feel to follow specific kinds of writing center orthodoxies, such as tutoring in specific modes (Nicklay, 2012). When tutors fail to follow the rules or fail to produce good feeling in and throughout the session (Giaimo et al., 2018), they struggle with all kinds of negative feelings, such as guilt, anxiety, embarrassment, and shame.

DEFINING AND IDENTIFYING EMOTIONAL LABOR IN WRITING CENTERS

Of course, emotional labor is a critical element of the work that writing centers perform. However, emotional labor is complicated because it comprises a mixture of the kinds of expectations that are placed knowingly upon workers as well as those workspace expectations that may be hidden and unspoken. In reviewing the scholarship on this subject, and in order to interrogate and name the emotional labor demanded of writing center workers, I have developed a set of discussion questions that can help WCAs and tutors to think deeply and broadly about the kinds of occupational expectations, particularly emotional ones, writing center work demands.

- What kinds of emotional labor do our jobs demand of us?
- What kinds of emotional labor do we, as WCAs, demand of tutors?
- What kinds of emotional labor do we, as WCAs, demand of ourselves?
- Which training modules explicitly try to manage workers' emotional activities?
- Which training modules implicitly try to manage workers' emotional activities?
- What kinds of emotional labor do we, as tutors, demand of other tutors?
- What kinds of emotional labor do we, as tutors, demand of our WCAs?
- What is my philosophy and approach for engaging with "the public"?
- Do I want to produce specific emotional states in other people at the Writing Center?
- What are my expectations for how people will feel when using the Writing Center?
- What motivates me to do writing center work?

TOWARD AN INCLUSIVE AND INTERSECTIONAL EMOTIONAL LABOR HEURISTIC IN WRITING CENTERS

While workplace expectations for performing emotional labor are hazardous when they are not fully articulated or described, there are other issues with expecting workers to perform this kind of labor.

One major issue, as I see it arising in Hochschild's research, is how bound-up emotional labor is with class, race, gender, and other circumstances that are particular to individual workers. The "commoditization of feeling may not have equal salience for all social classes" (Hochschild, 1979, p. 569); additionally, this kind of affective work is likely to fall to people from marginalized backgrounds, such as people of color (Evans & Moore, 2015) and women, regardless of whether it is articulated (and compensated) or not, especially in higher education (Schueths et al., 2013). Without articulating, interrogating, and ultimately compensating the emotional labor expectations attendant to writing center work, we run the risk of further exploiting people from marginalized backgrounds through expecting their participation in a largely unarticulated praxis of emotional labor. Therefore, in addition to defining, identifying, and discussing emotional labor in the writing center, it is critical to develop a plan wherein this work does not fall disproportionately to marginalized workers. So, in addition to diversifying writing centers' hiring practices, clear articulation of protective policies is critical in ameliorating any exploitative working conditions. Of course, the field ought to interrogate center hiring and workplace practices and develop ethical standards for writing center labor (Perdue et al., 2017).

Yet another issue regarding inclusion and emotional labor is how writing centers broadcast certain class-based assumptions through their hiring and training practices. Though the model has been critiqued (Denny et al., 2018; Faison, 2018), writing centers are largely framed as middle-class spaces (McKinney, 2005) or unclassed spaces. Yet, as Hochschild noted, emotional labor of the "toe" kind is often associated with service industries. Because they have been socialized to respond in particular ways to conflict, middle-class workers are groomed, and subsequently recruited, because they are adept at emotional regulation. Until we interrogate how writing centers interact with class—who feels belonging in the center and who does not—we cannot fully conceive of how emotional labor in writing centers can stand apart from suppression of negative thought and experience. Recent research on microaggressions in writing centers (Hermann, 2017), as well as research on anti-racism (Condon, 2007; Diab et al., 2012; García, 2017), can help us to walk the line between training staff to manage their emotions but not to demand they relinquish them in order to produce good feeling in clients. There must be a balance between these two competing imperatives—personal and public experiences of feeling—of emotional labor in writing center work.

BURNOUT AND EMOTIONAL LABOR

While research on emotional labor in writing centers is fairly well developed, research on burnout in writing centers is less developed. In her thesis, Rowell (2015) includes a section on burnout that heavily relies on Sherwood's (1995) "The Dark Side of the Helping Personality: Student Dependency and the Potential for Tutor Burnout," a chapter that "leads us to realize that by being too helpful to students, writing center practitioners risk burnout for themselves and dependency by the writers" (Strand, 1996, p. 11). Rowell argues that "there is potential for this burnout to be avoided and eliminated altogether" (p. 30). Relying on a number of recommendations from Sherwood (1995) that echo mindfulness practices, Rowell argues that tutors practice " 'enlightened self-interest' (p. 68) as well as 'detached concern' (p. 69) as some means of protection from burnout" (p. 30).

Burnout, however, is not just the pesky outcome of engaging in writing center labor; it is its own complex phenomenon, and it warrants attention that is separate from studying emotional labor. As Maslach et al. (2001) describe it, burnout is a response to "chronic emotional and interpersonal stressors on the job" (p. 397). There are three criteria to burnout: "A 'progressive loss of idealism, energy, and purpose experienced by people in the helping professions as a result of the conditions of their work' " (Sanchez-Reilly et al., 2013, p. 1). It is identifiable in workers by the following indicators:

- Physical and emotional exhaustion
- Cynicism
- Inefficacy

Burnout, then, results from unchecked emotional and other workplace stressors; therefore, it is critical to evaluate when emotional labor associated with a job shifts from manageable to unmanageable. Of course, the first step in evaluating what is manageable emotional labor is identifying the kinds of emotional labor that are performed and evaluating whether the workplace expectations for emotional labor are reasonable and workers are supported in undertaking this kind of work.

However, burnout is also its own separate issue. While unchecked and unexamined emotional labor might contribute to writing center workers experiencing burnout, there are other factors that contribute to this condition. Therefore, before trying to alleviate burnout, as Rowell suggests, it is critical to recognize the signs of burnout and to think about ways to confront burnout in writing center work. Of course, this involves the necessary confrontation of the neoliberal university (Monty, 2019) and its contribution to scarcity economics, which, in turn, contribute to burnout conditions experienced by workers and students alike.

WHAT STRUCTURAL LIMITATIONS AND LACK OF SUPPORT LEAD TO BURNOUT

In many ways, writing centers are spaces ripe for employee burnout; they are public-serving spaces that often labor under precarious financial conditions. They often have high employee turnover—by virtue of employing student and adjunct labor—and generally struggle, even within the broader field of rhetoric and composition, with legitimization issues. The field itself has an underdog history in which the "low status" of writing center work is often juxtaposed with love and deep commitment to writing center work (Geller & Denny, 2013). Generally speaking, our collective field has a chip on its shoulder for being less privileged and more service-and-administration-oriented than even our WPA counterparts. These issues trickle down into most facets of how we do our work—from how we train our staffs to how we administer and report on our labor.

Couple these field-specific issues with the rising precarity that higher education is experiencing more generally, and we have a perfect storm that can quickly lead to worker burnout. One major chronic workplace stressor that has a profound effect on workers is the kind of budgetary model that is in place. Working under austerity measures—as I did for years—leaves indelible marks upon the emotional psyches of workers. Couple these external financial pressures—which push centers to ever-further optimization of their workforces—with the emotional pressures that writing center workers feel to deliver positive feeling through writing center labor, and exploitation happens swiftly.

There was a time in my career when I always tried to do more with less. I naively thought that such thrift and restraint would be rewarded; my working-class upbringing, in this instance, shaped this philosophy, but so too did the logic of disaster capitalism. What I came to learn, however, is that the more you do with less, the more that is taken away from you. At least in a system where austerity measures are in place, a "thrift" model that encourages consistent growth places too much pressure on an already overextended labor force. WCAs need to think carefully about the kinds of managers they want to be and the kinds of goals they want their centers to develop and achieve. My experience "rehabbing" neglected writing centers has taught me that this work is often done on the backs of workers. This is not the only way; however, less exploitative approaches to writing center administration involve intentionality, planning, and patience. It also involves developing a personal managerial philosophy and ethos.

We are not really trained to think much about our management philosophies. In fact, we are often discouraged from framing our work within managerial terms; this is true even in writing center administration (Heckelman, 1998) and writing program administration (Strickland, 2011). In not framing our work within managerial contexts, however, it is easy to fall into unintentional behaviors that mimic the work habits of late-stage capitalism. Of course, working against the managerial framework also comes with its own hazards; in attempting to be democratic and nonhierarchical, we fail to account for and protect marginalized workers. No matter how much we attempt to decouple our work from management, the typical organizational issues that come from either weak or overbearing management will still arise. Therefore, it is critical to develop an intentional and ethical approach to management, which can help to mitigate burnout among staff, even if the center is housed in an institution that struggles with budgetary shortfalls and other precarity.

CONCLUSION

It is impossible for writing center labor—which is education work, and part of a helping profession—to be completely separated from emotional labor. In fact, the emotional labor that our field performs is a critical element to the support and confidence-building of generations of students (clients and workers alike) and encourages us to be inclusive and empowering spaces for underrepresented students at our colleges and universities. However, in failing to identify and explore the many different kinds of labor—including emotional labor—that writing center practitioners are expected to perform, we run the risk of under-preparing our workers for writing center work, which can lead to exploitation and other downstream negative effects. Additionally, such prolonged stressors can contribute to staff burnout, which goes along with dissatisfaction and attrition. And while tutors can utilize mindfulness strategies, as Rowell (2015) and Costello (2021) note, to describe and reflect upon the kinds of emotional labor that they perform, or feel compelled to perform, this work should not stop at the local level.

WCAs need to do more research on burnout and develop research-informed models of ethical administration and management. From my own research, especially the findings I share on tutors' experience of stress in Chapter 2, I learned that tutors often struggle to articulate nega-tive experiences with writing center work, perhaps because of the heavy investment they have in the writing center beyond seeing it as a work-place and a job. In discussing emotional labor, then, it is important to not create a coercive space that demands toxic positivity. Of course, we know that labor—and its attendant work stressors like burnout—affect workers from different identities in different ways. Yet without clear workplace expectations and protective policies, it is likely that the most marginalized among us will take on too much stress, engage in too much emotional labor, and, ultimately, will derive less satisfaction and positive outcomes from writing center work.

So, while my research is a preliminary foray into understanding the complex and multifaceted experiences of emotional labor and burnout among tutors, it is still preliminary. We need to know more about how tutors from different and marginalized backgrounds experience emo-tional labor and burnout. We need to learn more about how tutors from different socioeconomic backgrounds process—or fail to process—how emotions feature in their daily work experiences. In short, we need to learn more about how identity affects tutor engagement with emotional labor and experience of burnout. In the next chapter, I discuss systemic oppression and the complexities of labor issues that writing center workers from marginalized backgrounds face and share an anti-racist wellness heuristic rooted in Black liberation movements (civil rights, Black feminism) as part of a necessary corrective to these issues. The other part of this corrective, as I have argued here, relies on policies, protections, and anti-racist training, as much as it does recruitment and mentorship of underrepresented people into writing center work.

7

LOCATING WELLNESS IN BLACK LIBERATION SOCIAL MOVEMENTS
Toward an Anti-Racist Wellness Model in Writing Centers

OPENING NARRATIVE

As I have continued to explore and study wellness-related issues, I have come to realize the necessity of historically contextualizing and ethically implementing such interventions in the writing center. I have also come to believe that individualistic and bootstrapping approaches to wellness are part of a neoliberal agenda that minimizes institutional culpability while pressuring individuals to take action—often at their own personal expense. Alternatives to wellness structured around a white racial habitus recognize, among other things, the relationship between wellness and Black feminism. In recognizing this relationship, it is also necessary to call attention to the absence of any kind of sustained wellness research or articulated support plan on wellness interventions that explicitly support marginalized people—particularly Black people—in writing centers. In short, a lot of modern-day wellness scholarship—inside and outside writing center studies—draws upon a white habitus that denies or simply fails to locate its political, anti-materialist, altruistic, and activist origins. To challenge this kind of wellness—that is coopted and corporatized—I situate wellness practices in non-white, working-class, and non-Western spaces. In Chapter 4, I discussed the connection between modern mindfulness practices and Zen Buddhism. I have also talked about how class and gender are brought to bear on the wellness work we perform—or choose not to perform—in Chapter 6. Here, I talk about self-care, emotional labor, and other wellness issues as they relate to race, gender, and systemic oppression.

LITERATURE REVIEW
The Relationship Between Health, Well-Being, and Black Liberation
There have been multiple moments in the 20th century when wellness initiatives have intersected and overlapped with the medical industry.

https://doi.org/10.7330/9781646423606.c007

As Nelson (2015) notes, in 1948 the World Health Organization defined health as "a state of complete physical, mental and social well-being and not merely the absence of disease or infirmity" (p. 1). Yet it wasn't until after World War II that this more robust definition of health became popularized in the United States because of the work of social activists—civil rights activists first, then Black and white feminists. At this time, activists and scholars identified the intersection of political enfranchisement with well-being, physical health, and access to support. Systemic social issues, such as generational poverty and racism, profoundly affected health but, also, personal autonomy. During the Civil Rights Movement, "demands for basic needs made by everyday people living with Jim Crow" became a rallying call for community-engagement and support (p. 4). One of these basic needs, which was met by community organizers, was that of medical care. Activists and medical professionals, such as H. Jack Geiger, created community health centers that provided medical care to poor and undersupported people of color during Jim Crow.

The civil rights movement focused on redefining health alongside creating healthcare interventions that were acutely aware of white supremacy and that engaged "individuals and communities in their own health promotion" (p. 5). It is not surprising that health—broadly conceived—and wellness interventions were cornerstone issues of this movement, which aimed to liberate Black people, and people of color more broadly, from the systems of oppression that reached into most facets of their lived experience, because, as Nelson notes, "legal rights alone would do little to dismantle white supremacy" (p. 4).

However, "scientific sexism" (Ehrenreich & English, 2005, p. 13) against women—particularly women of color and working-class women—persisted even after the establishment of community healthcare centers during the civil rights movement (Nelson, 2015, p. 4). In the 1960s and 1970s, feminists continued to address systemic oppression through the medical and legal fields by advocating for reproductive and other healthcare rights; however, it was because of pressure from women of color that "eradication of socioeconomic barriers to health and reproductive autonomy [became] more central to a feminist political agenda" (p. 2). Arguments for "revolutionizing health care in order to transform social hierarchy," however, preceded second-wave feminism (p. 2). Nelson notes that "many of the women who became involved in the feminist movement first worked with these prior movements" such as the New Left movement and the civil rights movement (p. 2).

BLACK FEMINISM AND RADICAL CARE

The politics of care are critical to Black feminism (Collins, 1989; Nash, 2013). Black scholars and activists, perhaps most famously Audre Lorde (2017), but also including June Jordan (1995), bell hooks (2000), and Angela Davis (Afropunk, 2018) have written and spoken about the importance of self-care and self-love for Black women. Recently, Davis acknowledged the importance of self-care for Black activists who face all kinds of chronic illnesses and trauma related to their experiences of systemic oppression and murder, and who may also struggle to perform their activist work because of these traumas (Gorski, 2019). Lorde, in writing about her metastasized liver cancer, draws parallels between her "continuing battle for self-determination and survival" (p. 41), living with cancer, and the battle that "Black women fight daily, often in triumph" (p. 41). Lorde argues that her life has been prolonged because of the decision to "maintain some control over my life for as long as possible" (p. 40). Lorde argues that self-care, then, is a radical act of "self-preservation," that requires taking agency, which, because of the systemic oppression and devaluing of Black bodies—particularly Black women—becomes "an act of political warfare" (p. 130). In finding what is "joyful and life-affirming" (p. 131), despite her cancer, Lorde challenges our pathologizing of women who are ill, particularly Black and Brown women who are ill. Taylor (2018), echoing Lorde, argues for radical self-love that reconfigures how we perceive and feel about body difference. adrienne maree brown (2019) extends this work in *Pleasure Activism*, where she identifies pleasure as "a measure of freedom" and asks readers to reframe "scarcity thinking around the pursuit of pleasure" (p. 1). Pleasure activism, in this sense, seeks to reclaim pleasure as an activist and anti-racist pursuit. Lorde, Taylor, and brown flip common cultural figurations for Black women from tragedy and abjection to joy, empowerment, self-love, and pleasure.

WELLNESS SELF-CARE TRENDS IN POPULAR CONTEXTS

Popular and current models of self-care seem to run completely counter to the politically motivated and anti-racist approach that was taken by Black feminists. Wellness has become a modern-day self-help phenomenon and a booming multi-trillion-dollar industry (Global Wellness Institute, 2020). Several critiques have been lodged against the current figurations of wellness industries and culture, but chief among them is that modern-day wellness—particularly the radical Black feminist concept of self-care—has become divorced from its racial, political, and anti-racist origins (Spicer, 2019), and has instead become coopted and contorted to serve the neoliberal turn toward individualistic (and often white and upper-class) notions of care (DeRango-Adem, 2017; Harris, 2017; Mahdawi, 2017). Gunther (2018) further warns that in this iteration, the "wellness industrial complex" is trending toward melding its practices with pseudo-scientific fringe movements, such as those of anti-vaxxers. Therefore, wellness trends on social media and elsewhere are facilitating the political radicalization of people while also spreading anti-health conspiracy theories.

While there has been an explosion of politically hollow and individualistic wellness services (Kisner, 2017), around 2015 there was also an increased interest in wellness models that are robust, community-oriented, anti-racist, and focused on people of color. In part, this renewed interest in self-care stems from research that connects racism with intergenerational trauma, PTSD, and chronic health issues (Harrell et al., 2003; Berger & Sarnyai, 2015). A related "factor that has prompted renewed interest in self-care in the black community is the rise in media attention to police killings of unarmed black people" (Harris, 2017) and the emergence of the Black Lives Matter movement, which struggles with issues attendant to activist burnout and trauma (The Establishment, 2016; Mirk, 2016). As a new model of digital activism (and information sharing) has taken root, conversations have turned to how already-traumatized Black people navigate social media spaces full of violence against Black bodies. Research on racism and PTSD, as well as research on the deleterious effects of viewing violence in media regarding mental health (Busso et al., 2014; Adetiba & Almendrala, 2016; Williams & Delapp, 2016; Garza, 2020) have helped give shape to new conversations about Black activism and self-care.

Additionally, there are several nonacademic community wellness organizations and online communities that utilize social media and online environments to promote sustainable, politically engaged, and BIPOC-focused wellness services. Frequently, these organizations and collectives are founded upon and deliberately reference racial justice movements of the mid-20th century. One such community, GirlTrek, specifically honors and refers to the civil rights movement—and the chronic health issues that the Black community faces—on their website: "In the footsteps of a civil rights legacy, GirlTrek is a national health movement that activates thousands of Black women to be change makers in their lives and communities—through walking." GirlTrek engages in community-oriented healthcare initiatives focused on empowerment and agency-building specifically focused on self-care and women's healing (McCabe, 2020), which is a far cry from the tepid wellness industrial complex focused on individuals and expensive services rather than community-oriented political action.

Another wellness space focused on supporting marginalized people but, also, necessarily offering community engagement is Body Politic—a "Queer Feminist Wellness Collective, Event Series, and Media Company." While Body Politic was established recently (2018), it intentionally combines business support for wellness initiatives alongside a feminist collective ethos that provides mutual aid and other kinds of support. One of its main missions is to "serve marginalized communities and groups that have typically been left out of the wellness conversation." One initiative from this collective is a publication, *Body Type*, that writes about "underdiscussed issues in wellness—the ways wellness intersects with issues like sexuality, race, gender, size, ability, financial accessibility, and more." It promises to be an alternative to "commoditized wellness space[s]." And, since March 2020, when the collective's founder and its artistic director both contracted COVID-19, Body Politic has also become a gathering space, information clearing house, and support network for young people who have contracted the virus and many of whom have struggled with long-term and chronic effects of becoming ill (Lowenstein, 2020).

Digital technologies can enable the proliferation of community-oriented spaces that advance rhetorically complex, savvy, and activist-oriented wellness initiatives. One example of this is Afropunk's "Radical Self-Care Week," which advocates for explicit acts of self-care by Black people. As Satya (2019) notes,

> Radical Self Care may be a trend, but it's one of the best trends that has ever happened to Black people. The idea of Black people taking back control over their own minds, bodies and spirits is exactly what's needed to survive in a system that constantly tells us that our wellness isn't important. Self care is a radical act because, let's be honest, sometimes it's easier to take care of everyone else except ourselves. Black people have been indoctrinated to believe that they should put themselves last—but putting ourselves first is key. (n.p.)

Afropunk (2018) also shared a video on self-care and activism featuring Angela Davis. In the video, Davis talks about the importance of self-care—and mindfulness—particularly for BIPOC activists. In telling a story about Black Panther leader Ericka Huggins, who began practicing yoga and meditation—and who urged other Panthers like Bobby Seale to do so as well—Davis talks about how wellness interventions can be critical tools to fight burnout, fatigue, PTSD, and other adverse effects of systemic racism, which are particularly damaging to political activists. Davis acknowledges her own practice of yoga and meditation while incarcerated, though she realizes the importance of the collective in engaging in such practices.

A final example comes from a local wellness intervention that recently occurred in a workplace. A Haitian restaurant in Brooklyn, Grandchamps, arranged a discussion with a Haitian human rights lawyer on the topic of racial profiling and being stopped by the police (Estrin, 2020). The owners of the restaurant were responding both to the current pandemic as well as the recent (but ongoing) BLM protests of the murders of Black people (George Floyd and Breonna Taylor, among others) by the police. Because these protests brought out a large police presence in New York City, and because the majority of the restaurant's workers had been stopped by the police at one point or another, many workers felt fear over being stopped on their way to or from work. Their discussion aimed to address "the practical and emotional consequences of a moment when the Black community is being disproportionately affected by the coronavirus, and as protests against police violence dredge up memories and anxieties of their own experiences with law enforcement" (Estrin, 2020). One of the restaurant owners, Ms. Brockman, identified her desire for Black people to thrive even during such a chaotic and dangerous moment. The other owner, Shawn Brockman, purposely wants to change restaurant culture, where disrespectful and aggressive behavior is common in the workplace.

These are just a few examples culled from the media, popular press, and digital spaces in which wellness intersects with race, gender, and class. These grassroots initiatives, which are located outside of the academy and are not yet featured within it, locate wellness within historical, political, and anti-racist frameworks. Many of these wellness initiatives are aimed at millennials and Gen Z-ers; however, they also acknowledge the previous dearth of intentional, collective, politically oriented wellness initiatives, especially for Black people and people from other marginalized identities. I offer these as some of the best that wellness initiatives can provide to communities—especially within academia—that are hungry for recognition, engagement, and support. Since millennials and Gen Z-ers (who now comprise a large cross-section of the student-tutor population in American colleges and universities) are the ones driving many of these anti-racist wellness initiatives, I doubt that these groups will be resistant to acknowledging the need for intersectional and community-oriented wellness initiatives. I do, however, think it is important to elevate the work of wellness (and self-care) as politically impactful, inclusive, and rooted in movements for and about Black people, and especially Black women; I am not sure that this connection is readily apparent to cis white people given how thoroughly assimilated and commodified the wellness industrial complex has become. In acknowledging and exploring the intersection between Black liberation, wellness, and current anti-racist activism, practitioners can begin to develop sustainable anti-racist heuristics for wellness that are locally situated but collectively (and perhaps digitally) structured. Such centering of wellness within anti-racist and activist movements is critical for reimagining workplaces comprised of marginalized workers.

Of course, the stakes of such wellness work can be life and death: In January 2020, Shawnton Clay—a team organizer for GirlTrek—was murdered (Alund, 2020). The founder of Body Politic contracted COVID-19 and almost died. Employees at Grandchamps were harassed and detained by the police. Wellness work taking place in the private and public sectors around the country can also be activist work. Black women, queer women, and others who do this work also struggle with health and other precarities. The link between wellness and anti-racism is, unfortunately, left largely unexplored in current published research in the field of writing center studies; therefore, it is necessary to do the extra connective work with writing center workers and to recognize that racism produces PTSD and generational trauma, which is deleterious to the health and wellbeing of Black people (Black et al., 2015). However, situating wellness in health (and the body as much as the mind) can also allow WCAs to address the unique needs of marginalized people in our centers and, perhaps, establish community support networks to do so.

WRITING CENTERS, RACE, AND WELLNESS

While writing center studies has a history of engagement with wellness studies and wellness interventions (Gamache, 2003; Murray, 2003; Spohrer, 2008) that span over 20 years, it is only in the past few years that wellness research has been reconnected to its origins in Black feminism and addressed racism. A number of recently published articles (Faison & Treviño, 2017; Green, 2018; Faison, 2019; Haltiwanger Morrison & Nanton, 2019) by Black and Latinx women articulate experiences of racism in writing centers and argue for radical acts of naming but, also, reexamination of "safe spaces" within anti-racist contexts.

These scholars identify a fundamental issue with writing centers, which is that they occupy a white, middle-class habitus (often centered around white feminism and white liberal values) that excludes people—especially workers—from marginalized backgrounds (Haltiwanger Morrison & Nanton, 2019). For those tutors that are outside of that habitus, writing centers are not welcoming, or especially safe, spaces. The current deployment of wellness rhetoric and wellness interventions in writing centers is often bolstered by this habitus. In reconnecting wellness to anti-racist and explicitly Black feminist activism, these scholars uncover a critical but missing piece of doing wellness work. Divorced from its radical roots, wellness becomes a cudgel that, in the name of civility and other middle-class notions of politeness, is used to police the behaviors of people of color. Talia Nanton (Haltiwanger Morrison & Nanton, 2019) shares personal experiences of working as an undergraduate in a writing center that reveal this cooptation of wellness work toward purposes that silence and alienate people of color, particularly Black women, in writing centers. She writes:

> As a Black woman, I was called "aggressive" by a peer and accused of "creating tension" and taking conversations "out of hand" when I stuck up for myself in debates where it seemed as though the opinions of others were welcome but not my own. I was reprimanded for being disrespectful after not saying "hello" to another co-worker, however unintentionally, all under the guise of making sure the center remained "a safe space." I was berated for the actions of other consultants, such as playing music too loud, and accused of not taking criticism well. (2019)

Nanton recounts a series of experiences of how, as a Black woman, she was treated differently from her white peers. Her behavior was policed. She was not given the benefit of the doubt regarding her actions. She was blamed for others' behaviors. Her affect and her ideas were silenced. Her behaviors and emotions were viewed as threatening and were criticized. I summarize—rather than interpret—these experiences because I do not want to detract from the daily and numerous injustices that Black women face when they enter predominately white spaces. Nanton (Haltiwanger Morrison & Nanton, 2019) identifies how policing and bodily control within the space help to preserve the writing center's white, middle-class habitus and faux-inclusive spaces; white people's comfort, in this instance, takes precedence over a Black woman's safety. Nanton was punished for speaking out about her experiences with racism in the center, as she notes, "under the guise of making sure the center remained 'a safe space'" (2019, n.p.). While the use of the term "safe space" here might seem like it is divorced from wellness—or, at the least, being raised in the hope of tutors' well-being, I see the use of this term as coercive in that it manages and silences the emotional and lived experiences of a Black tutor. The safe space, then, becomes the surveillance and policing mechanism that white management utilizes to dictate what emotions and interpersonal engagements are allowed in the workplace.

As I am sure most WCAs will agree, this is *not* how we want tutors—particularly tutors of color—to experience writing center work. In response to Nanton's experience, Talisha Haltiwanger Morrison (Haltiwanter Morrison & Nanton, 2019) suggests that writing centers are underprepared for supporting people who fall outside of the white, middle-class habitus: "I think what those in writing centers must realize is that one of the reasons we must work not to harm our students, tutors, colleagues, and others, is that we are not working with blank slates. This is not the first time you in particular or Black women in general have been made to feel unwelcome. It's simply a new context." Calling attention to the effects of systemic racism, Haltiwanger Morrison points to the importance of recognizing what people of color bring into the center. In other words, "The racism Black people experience in the writing center isn't isolated from other experiences of racism" (Haltiwanger Morrison & Nanton, 2019).

Additionally, writing centers, by virtue of being predominately liberal spaces that rely on white feminist notions of inclusion, have failed to genuinely confront racism and the kinds of discrimination people of color experience in this space. Haltiwanger Morrison and Nanton (2019) note:

> As for the idea of White feminism, and how it fails Black women, it reflects this framework of appearing so "open" and forward, to the point where other voices are being silenced because they become unfathomable in the space. I definitely believe that my female director, like so many White feminists, or even liberal White Americans, fail to realize their own racism and the role they have in reinforcing oppressive structures primarily because they also fail to consider how they may need to continue discussions on racism and how it exists within a variety of forms and within many, if not all, institutions, as well as realizing that those discussions cannot only be held solely amongst themselves and without real inclusivity.

Haltiwanger Morrison and Nanton (2019) and others (Faison & Treviño, 2017; Faison, 2019) rightly identify that there is a lot more work to do in deconstructing white, middle-class habitus in writing centers and becoming genuinely inclusive spaces for people of color. Instead of instituting monolithic wellness programs that are predicated on white feminist (or worse, neoliberal) values, therefore, we need to interrogate "the connections between forms of oppression"

(Haltiwanger Morrison & Nanton, 2019) and create targeted and specialized wellness interventions with that knowledge—and the knowledge of generational trauma—in mind. And, also, we need to examine how "safe spaces" might uphold a white, middle-class habitus that elevates respectability and consensus-building at the expense of the experiences and ideas of people of color. In this way, we need to interrogate our own internalized racism and actively question *why* consensus, harmony, or other "safe" forms of communication are ones writing centers seem to hew toward.

I want to recognize that many of the articles I am discussing in this section recount numerous moments when individual tutors and administrators of color—many of whom are Black women—experienced discrimination from co-workers, WCAs, and clients. These women also experienced non-belonging within writing centers, some of which stemmed from writing centers' focus on white, upper-middle-class aesthetics (Faison & Treviño, 2017), which articulated "raced and classed hierarchies with its performance of domestic life and its presupposed upper middle-class domestic comforts" (Faison, 2019, p. 53). Some scholars, such as Green (2018) and Nanton (Haltiwanger Morrison & Nanton, 2019), detail countless experiences of discrimination and microaggressions. While white directors and tutors might with all good intentions be quick to argue that inclusion is a critical cornerstone of most writing center philosophies, it is critical that we interrogate who feels inclusion and belonging in writing center spaces.

In rushing to create harmonious spaces, informed by white, middle-class aesthetics and politics, we risk speaking over and negating the voices of writing center workers that come from other backgrounds. Perhaps unsurprisingly, this dynamic is one that was played out by white feminists during second-wave feminism—with white feminists ignoring and negating Black and Brown feminists' experiences of oppression; therefore, we need to recognize where writing centers' current figurations of inclusion come from—such as white feminism and other white liberal political movements—and reorient toward more fitting activist movements and away from ones that have failed women/people of color. Because anti-racist work is ongoing and requires continual engagement, and because of the connections between wellness and anti-racist work, I provide a set of anti-racist wellness interventions actions that writing center administrators can implement in their centers. Most of these interventions were informed by the scholarship and/or experiences of women scholars of color, from the field of writing center studies as well as Black feminist studies.

ANTI-RACIST WELLNESS INTERVENTIONS
IN THE WRITING CENTER

- Acknowledge and discuss the origins of wellness interventions in social justice movements, such as Black liberation and feminism (self-care) as well as in spiritual practices, such as Buddhism (mindfulness).

- "Acknowledge your privilege, and be willing to give some of it up" (Haltiwanger Morrison & Nanton, 2019, citing Green, 2018).

- Consider "the experiences of POC [as] both valid and measurable" (Faison & Treviño, 2017). Avoid gaslighting people who experience discrimination.

- Work against a neoliberal configuration of wellness in which the interventions are in place to optimize, coerce, and exploit (rather than interrogate and reconfigure) labor.

- Understand the connections between racism and trauma and account for these connections when developing policies and expectations around engaging with wellness (refrain from forcing or otherwise making these interventions mandatory).

- Value "those experiences of POC within a cultural context" (Faison & Treviño, 2017).

- Recognize that wellness will be engaged with, performed, and even conceptualized differently by different people—do not impose only a white, middle-class habitus on wellness programs.

- Leave space for people of color to share their experiences but, also, to not share their experiences with wellness.

- Discuss the physiological as well as the psychological effects of stress and account for the interconnection of the mind/body in wellness practices.

- Engage in positive affirmation of workers (and each other) in the center.

- In some systemic way, interrogate your writing center's culture and who feels belonging in the space. Haltiwanger Morrison and Nanton (2019) suggest "conducting a case-study on your center's 'safe-ness.' "

- Interrogate your writing center's policies and the impact they have on staff members, particularly from marginalized backgrounds.

- Interrogate why and how your writing center reprimands workers.

- Interrogate center hierarchies and workplace expectations—are workers of color represented in leadership roles? Are workers of color doing more work than nonmarginalized (white) workers?

- Create flexible work policies that consider workers' physical and mental health. Learn about intergenerational trauma and chronic PTSD among marginalized populations.

- Where possible, cultivate a community-oriented (rather than solely individualistic) wellness model.

- Where possible, provide resources for Black women and other people of color on self-care, such as http://www.poconlineclassroom .com/self-care and https://thefeministwire.com/2014/04/self-love -and-self-care and http://www.bellhooksinstitute.com/welcome.

- Where possible, provide resources on anti-racism to white people in the center https://advisingcorps.org/antiracism/ and https:// education.uconn.edu/anti-racism-resources-for-students-educators -and-citizens and https://facultydevelopment.cornell.edu/anti -racism.

- "Have open dialogue about microaggressions, discrimination, and racism—create time for informal check-ins with tutors (being open and accessible to discuss issues in the center)" (Haltiwanger Morrison & Nanton, 2019).

- Don't assume that racism and other types of discrimination cannot happen in your writing center.

- Have open dialogues about center practices and whether they uphold "oppressive ideologies" (Faison & Treviño, 2017), which, for marginalized tutors, can be painful to enforce.

- Conduct "research that focuses on the experiences of historically marginalized bodies working and receiving assistance/services in the WC" (Faison & Treviño, 2017).

- Institute "implicit bias training for all staff, including tutors of color" (Haltiwanger Morrison & Nanton, 2019).

- Rely on "the voices and experiences of tutors of color to inform the practices and scholarship of our field" (Haltiwanger Morrison & Nanton, 2019).

CONCLUSION

As Faison and Treviño (2017) note, retention of marginalized people as writing center workers is difficult work and, often, writing centers fail to do so, despite their best intentions. The changes I advocate in this chapter recognize that hiring more people of color and diversifying staff is simply not enough; as Haltiwanger Morrison and Nanton (2019) note, "Numbers on staff do not mean inclusion in a community or a sense of safety or welcomeness." Because neoliberal institutions do little to recruit or retain these populations, writing centers must take up the call to do deliberate anti-racist work, which necessarily means account-ing for the health and well-being of tutors of color in addition to greater attention paid toward how marginalized people move through writing center spaces. Here, the Civil Rights Movement and the Black feminist movement make apparent how critically intertwined the dismantling of racism is with access to basic needs, such as access to care and access to non-racist workspaces and other spaces. The list of interventions that

I provide, however, is a partial one and one that I have developed—in large part—*after* conducting research and assessment on the wellness interventions instituted in my writing center and *after* listening to tutors and graduate administrators—many of whom were from marginalized backgrounds. Anti-racist work is ongoing and we will not always get it "right" when we try to implement it within our centers. But, as a working-class first-generation queer person, I feel it is not only my responsibility to recruit and retain a more diverse group of tutors but also that these tutors should *thrive* in their work.

To that end, in order to undertake an anti-racist wellness (or other) project in a writing center, it is critical to gather stakeholders together and to listen to their experiences, and, if they are willing to share them, grievances. There is, of course, often an unfair onus placed upon people of color to articulate their experiences of oppression and racism. To avoid this toxic dynamic—with people of color doing the work to make unsafe spaces safer for them through education and "performing" their oppression—people from less marginalized backgrounds need to do this work. This means promoting self-education and group discussion among less marginalized people and listening, should marginalized workers want to speak. Dismantling white supremacist structures—particularly within racist institutions—is hard and long-term work. The first step, as I see it, involves refuting neoliberal models of wellness, which often encourage individualistic and relatively shallow care models, in favor of radical, anti-racist, and communal Black feminist ones.

Conclusion

THE FUTURE OF WELLNESS IN WRITING CENTER WORK

Wellness is complicated. It is a complex nexus of attitudes, philosophies, values, and practices that originate in Buddhism, the civil rights movement, and Black feminism; therefore, it is intersectional, interdisciplinary, political, revolutionary, and fundamentally anti-capitalist. Wellness is also part of a commercialized and depoliticized industry that is incredibly lucrative. There is a competing impulse between the capitalistic and optimization-focused wellness initiatives that are common in many types of institutional settings and the politically revolutionary wellness initiatives embraced by BLM activists and other grassroots and anti-materialist collectives. So, in addition to wellness being a complexly developed and enacted phenomenon, it is also a contradictory one that captures our current zeitgeist, insofar as it bolsters capitalism through productivity-oriented interventions while critiquing the very systems that it has been put in place to protect and support. Wellness, I feel I need to say again, is complicated! This book advocates for upending hegemonic uses of wellness and recognizing the important role such interventions can play in developing anti-racist and pro-labor workplaces.

I see the ways that wellness is deployed for both capitalistic and revolutionary ends on stark display in workplace wellness initiatives. From one vantage point, these initiatives are responding to just how unwell workplaces currently are for the average American worker. Informed by data on work-related stress, these wellness initiatives are responding to a widespread, chronic issue that affects a third of working Americans, yet they are put into place retroactively to combat the effects of workplace stress—chronic physical and mental illness among other adverse outcomes—without addressing the root causes of these symptoms, such as overwork and stagnant wages. Rather than identifying and mitigating the dynamics that create work stress—and all the attendant issues that come along with them—these wellness initiatives are retrofitted into the workplace as post hoc compensatory measures. So, while the unwell

https://doi.org/10.7330/9781646423606.c008

workplace is recognized by corporations and other businesses, wellness programs are enacted mainly on the back end to save these entities from the astronomical costs associated with the long-term effects of work-related stress. Through enacting such wellness programs, then, corporations both acknowledge and uphold the oppressive systems that are created by late-stage capitalism such as precarity, chronic stress, mental and physical health issues, and despair.

The higher-education industry, make no mistake, does not escape the fate of late-stage capitalism; it is also unwell. Adjunct and contingent labor and the dismantling of the tenure system are just a few of the trends in higher education that we currently face. In writing centers, more specifically, we struggle with the downstream effects of austerity in the neoliberal institution that eat away at our budgets while heaping more responsibilities upon us and while also attempting to support some of the most precarious enrollees at our institutions. Additionally, because many of our centers employ undergraduate and graduate students, or adjunct and staff workers, writing centers contain populations that face a complex set of wellness needs due to their employment precarity.

Wellness issues, then, have tendrils that reach into our working lives but also our personal lives. As the chapters on workplace stress, emergency planning and crisis response, emotional labor and burnout, and anti-racist wellness work all indicate, the writing center is not a bounded space where people enter and leave their troubles behind. It is also not a space that is value-neutral; the lived experiences of the people who make up the writing center staff are affected by racist, ableist, and otherwise oppressive institutional and government policies that make their way into the center. Because of all the ways in which systemic oppression, governmental policy, and violence affects institutions of higher learning, we face a growing set of wellness-related issues that demand our field's attention and our compassionate interventions. In particular, the growing instances of diagnosed and self-diagnosed mental health concerns (Degner et al., 2015) show that we must not only train our tutors in supporting and working with people who are distressed but also acknowledge and support workers struggling with mental health concerns. The rising rates of school shootings, and other on-campus aggressor situations, demonstrate the need for developing emergency plans that account for local contexts alongside identification of the potential hazards and risks that go along with working in (and attending) a writing center. Finally, the instances of police brutality and murder of people of color—particularly Black people—show us that we need to rethink how writing centers engage with campus and other police forces. But we also need to grapple with the long-term effects of racism on people of color who both utilize and work in the writing center. This means we need to establish deliberately anti-racist wellness training and support programs for center workers.

Part of this anti-racist wellness work is recuperative, insofar as our field acknowledges and learns about the work of Black scholars and Black activists who, during different social movements throughout the 20th and 21st centuries, advocated for more robust definitions of health that included wellness issues, such as access to physical and mental health support, empowerment to make health-related decisions, and community-focused and -centered care work. However, in addition to this recuperative component, anti-racist wellness work is also political. The radical reframing of care work as communal, political, and rooted in defiance of white supremacy (and attendant economic oppression) helps us to reorient wellness work away from productivity-oriented workplace models and toward an inclusive and radical reimagining of writing center workplaces.

We also need to do more wellness research in writing centers. Currently, wellness research—especially workplace wellness research—arises out of contradictory motivations to revolutionize work while optimizing labor and minimizing costs by placing the burden of care work onto individuals. As an example of this, Stoewen (2017) argues that veterinarians are ethically obligated to attend to their well-being and health because of the adverse effects lack of care has on patient outcomes (p. 861). Such tethering of personal obligations to optimize one's labor to the ethos of ethics obscures the large-scale and systemic issues that contribute to workers' lack of well-being. In connecting the individual's responsibility of being well to some kind of ethical code of conduct, a new and even more coercive optimization model is created. Now, one does not need to be well only for their companies and managers but also for their clients. In this model of wellness, the pressure and responsibility to be well is truly on the worker. Because writing centers have done relatively little work in wellness, we know little about whether our workplaces are coercive—though I imagine they are—and what kinds of pressures we put onto workers to be well while they work. The topic's relative newness in our field provides us with an opportunity to examine and potentially critique our current labor practices and to create our own exigencies for worker wellness and well-being that embrace anti-racist and fair-labor philosophies and practices.

It is also important to acknowledge and examine the kind of work that we do in educational settings. Writing center work is part of a "helping profession"; therefore, a lot of issues related to burnout creep into our centers, perhaps even when we believe we are doing everything we can to stave off such effects. As other helping professions have done, we need to develop a body of research—qualitative, quantitative, narratological, etc.—about how people in our field *work*. This should not be limited to those who have the most (although, often not much) staying power in the organization, such as WCAs, but also the undergraduate, graduate, adjunct, staff, and professional tutors that make up much of the writing center workforce. To start researchers on this journey, I hope that Chapter 3 will help new and more seasoned scholars to develop and carry out such labor-based projects.

Of course, a few years ago, the issues covered in this book—especially emergency planning—may have seemed just too far outside the purview of writing center workers (or educational workers more broadly) to be published. With the recent worldwide pandemic, however, such issues are palpable. Many of us were caught off guard when we had to shut down our centers, turn to remote tutoring, and engage in endless rounds of institutional planning (to re-open the colleges and universities, to prepare our spaces for in-person tutoring, to workforce- and budget-planning). COVID-19 has laid bare how deeply intertwined our institutions are with economic forces and precarity. The devil's bargain of always operating just at the margins—of profitability, of reach, of support—ensures that when crises hit, not only are we caught off guard, but our institutions turn quickly to austerity measures even as they endanger their workers' lives. The free-for-all fall 2020 semester—and the déjà vu of subsequent pandemic semesters—showed us that when pushed to make the decision between economic viability and worker wellness, most institutions choose money over safety and wellbeing of workers. So, while this book argues that writing centers ought to be prepared for any number of ways in which the wellness of its workers (and clients) are threatened, I also acknowledge that economics often trumps fair and safe workplace policies. This puts middle management (like WCAs) into the unfortunate position of having to choose between workers' wellness and workers' labor.

The situation that I am describing is no longer theoretical. COVID-19 has put on national display the conflict that millions of workers face choosing between safety and wellness and their economic livelihood. Again, writing centers are not exempt from making these moral (or immoral, as it were) calculations. Conversations on listservs, social media, and webinars during the first year and a half of the pandemic were largely centered on making the decision between in-person and virtual tutoring (or offering both services). Even as hospitalization rates soared, and daily reports brought record-topping infection rates, many of us tried to figure out how to accommodate the demands of the institution alongside the need to care for our workers. While the long arc of justice may eventually bend toward what is right, it is critical for everyday workers to make the decision to choose wellness over wealth-accumulation, because most institutions will not make the right or moral choice. This more ethical approach to decision-making, of course, would be made easier by having collective bargaining, union representation, and strong professional leadership. For my part, I helped reestablish a chapter of the American Association of University Professors (AAUP) at my institution that advocates for staff workers alongside faculty workers. I also broadly share professional guidelines for responding to COVID-19, such as the Conference on College Composition and Communication and Council of Writing Program Administrators joint statement on COVID-19 and remote teaching (CCCC & CWPA, 2020). Despite efforts such as these, there is much work to be done in our profession—and in higher education more broadly—to establish workplace conditions that are equitable, just, and attendant to our wellbeing.

Over time, perhaps, we will adjust to a new normal, though I hope we do not become complacent. At the moment, there are a range of conversations and actions taking place around wellness and labor issues in a number of different industries, including the helping professions, particularly higher education (Giaimo, 2020). The pandemic has brought into sharp relief just how badly workers are faring in the hyper-capitalist America of the early 21st century; this is a reality that we need to confront even as the "Great Resignation," or exodus of workers from the American marketplace, is hitting us in the face alongside unionization pushes reaching a fever pitch across the United States. Among many other industries, undergraduate student workers are unionizing and striking for better wages and safer workplaces on college campuses (Fitzpatrick, 2021). It is my hope that these movements for hazard and "hero" pay, drawing from governmental rainy day funds, drawing from swollen college endowments to shore up the most precarious workers and citizens, and unionization continue to gain momentum. In our field, I hope that we have conversations about how we labor in crises and what role writing centers can play during such cultural and economic flashpoints. This moment should lead to broader questions about the state of workers and work in writing centers. This moment should be one of institutional and organizational self-examination.

I want to end on a positive note. When I started integrating wellness and care work into my writing center management, I was doing so instinctually. I knew there were a complex set of factors contributing to the various "unwell" centers that I stepped into, factors that were related to underprofessionalization and other unclear workplace opportunities and guidelines; however, there were other forces like systemic racism, institutional precarity, and workplace burnout that I was only just beginning to grapple with. After switching jobs a few times, and seeing similar issues crop up in vastly different institutional contexts, I have come to realize that the work of one person could not fix these complex issues. In this way, my research work on wellness has helped me to take perspective and "know when to hold 'em, know when to fold 'em, know when to walk away, and know when to run," as Kenny Rogers (1978) sang. These experiences have shaped my administrative identity. But, contrary to the song, this is not the motto of a gambler. In fact, I have become more cautious and more adverse to risk as I have continued to integrate wellness training and support into my writing centers, because, in the end, I realize that even if my organizational structure adds only a few additional risks, or a few hazards, to workers' everyday experiences, they are still grappling with all the risks and hazards *outside* the writing center, as well as a number within the center that I cannot, under most circumstances, control. So, in this way, I have changed my administrative philosophy and, in the process, tried to chart a more moral and engaged path that not only accounts for workers' professional development but also their mental and physical wellbeing in their writing center work. Due to this work, I have been developing my own "personal systems of integrity" (Carter-Tod, 2020, p. 209) to lead my writing center but also represent the work I do to my broader academic community. I believe we can all do this work and I hope this book can be a compass that guides others as well.

I know, however, that this process is a messy and time-consuming one, but, as my research on attitudinal and cultural shifts toward workplace wellness interventions suggests, change does happen over time. My research assessment was developed during my journey to incorporate wellness into my writing centers. Now, this work has expanded out to include anti-racist work, anti-capitalist and labor-advocacy work, and more specific and bounded wellness interventions and policies in the writing center. So, yes, this is a messy but very rewarding process, and one that I hope can model for other writing center practitioners how to imagine better and more just futures for their workplaces that incorporate wellness theory and praxis from a wide variety of disciplines, philosophies, and social movements. We owe it to tutors, who are the lifeblood of writing centers, to do better and more engaged labor advocacy work that is anti-racist, anti-capitalist, and rooted in preserving peoples' dignity and wellness. We owe it to ourselves.

APPENDIX A

SAMPLE WELLNESS TRAININGS AT OSU 2016–2019

_____ August 2016 discussion Degner et al., "Opening Closed Doors: A Rationale for Creating a Safe Space for Tutors Struggling with Mental Health Concerns or Illnesses."

_____ September 2016, Group A mentorship, wellness ambassador training

_____ September 2016, Group B mentorship, wellness ambassador training

_____ September 2016, Group C mentorship, wellness ambassador training

_____ September 2016, Group D mentorship, wellness ambassador training

_____ Discussion and review of the "Guide to Assist Disruptive or Distressed Individuals," posted in Smith Lab writing center, or circulated via online link

_____ October 2016 all-staff meeting REACH suicide prevention presentation

_____ January 2017 training, active listening in the writing center

---

_____ August 2017 training, emergency and disaster planning

_____ August 2017 training, mindfulness and self-care in the Writing Center: Wellness Matters

_____ Group A mentorship, mindfulness training

_____ Group B mentorship, mindfulness training

_____ Group C mentorship, mindfulness training

_____ Group D mentorship, mindfulness training

_____ Discussion and review of the "Guide to Assist Disruptive or Distressed Individuals," posted in Smith lab writing center, or circulated via online link

_____ January 2018 training, emotional labor in the writing center

---

_____ August 2018 training, emergency and disaster planning

_____ August 2018 training, Community Wellness in WC training

_____ Group A mentorship, mindfulness training

_____ Group B mentorship, mindfulness training

_____ Group C mentorship, mindfulness training

_____ Group D mentorship, mindfulness training

_____ Group E mentorship, mindfulness training

_____ October 2018 all-staff meeting REACH suicide prevention presentation

_____ March 2019 Wellness and Self-Care All-Staff Meeting #3

https://doi.org/10.7330/9781646423606.c009

APPENDIX B

WRITING CENTER WELLNESS SURVEY (2016–2017)

PREAMBLE

The writing center is assessing its wellness-training efficacy, which is part of our on-going mission to provide support resources for consultants, clients, and the OSU community, more broadly. By taking this survey, you will help us develop new trainings, professionalization workshops, and mentorship group themes that focus on wellness. You will also help us to contribute vital research on the topic of wellness consultant support to the field of writing center studies. The survey is completely anonymous and you can stop at any point in the process of filling it out. This survey is not an evaluation of your mental state. If you experience stress while taking the survey, please seek counseling through OSU Counseling and Consultation Services, contact info: 1640 Neil Ave, Columbus, OH 43201, Phone: (614) 292-5766.

Please read each question and take careful consideration, as you complete the form.

I. Demographic Information

Graduate ___
Undergraduate ____
Short Response:
Academic department/major _____

II. Reflections on Your Well-Being:

1. I am capable of coping with my daily stress:

1	2	3	4	5
rarely	sometimes	often	mostly	always

2. I am able to appropriately manage my feelings:

1	2	3	4	5
rarely	sometimes	often	mostly	always

https://doi.org/10.7330/9781646423606.c010

3. I have positive relationships with colleagues, friends and/or family members:

1	2	3	4	5
Strongly Disagree	Disagree	Neutral	Agree	Strongly Agree

4. I have a colleague, friend and/or family member I can confide in:

1	2	3	4	5
rarely	sometimes	often	mostly	always

III. Effects of Recent Events on Campus

1. How much have you been concerned by the knife attack on campus?

1	2	3	4	5
Extremely	Significantly	Moderately	A little	Not at all

2. How much have you been concerned by the presidential election and current administration?

1	2	3	4	5
Extremely	Significantly	Moderately	A little	Not at all

3. How much have you been affected by the death of OSU student Reagan Tokes?

1	2	3	4	5
Extremely	Significantly	Moderately	A little	Not at all

How much have you been affected by the posting of racist and anti-diversity flyers on campus?

1	2	3	4	5
Extremely	Significantly	Moderately	A little	Not at all

4. I am confident handling unanticipated stressful events in the WC:

1	2	3	4	5
Strongly Disagree	Disagree	Neutral	Agree	Strongly Agree

5. How much have you been affected by the posting of anti-Trump flyers on campus?

1	2	3	4	5
Extremely	Significantly	Moderately	A little	Not at all

IV. Wellness Training Participation:

Please identify the wellness development opportunities that you participated in last semester (please select all that apply):

____ August 2016 discussion Degner et al., "Opening Closed Doors: A Rationale for Creating a Safe Space for Tutors Struggling with Mental Health Concerns or Illnesses."

____ September 2016, Group A (name redacted) mentorship, wellness ambassador training

____ September 2016, Group B (name redacted) mentorship, wellness ambassador training

____ September 2016, Group C (name redacted) mentorship, wellness ambassador training

____ September 2016, Group D (name redacted) mentorship, wellness ambassador training

____ Discussion and review of the "Guide to Assist Disruptive or Distressed Individuals," posted in Smith lab writing center, or circulated via online link

____ October 2016 all-staff meeting REACH suicide prevention presentation

____ January 2017 training, active listening in the writing center

V. Reflections on Your Wellness Training:

1. My wellness training has prepared me to handle stressful events in the Writing Center:

1	2	3	4	5
Strongly Disagree	Disagree	Neutral	Agree	Strongly Agree

2. My wellness training has helped me to support colleagues at the writing center:

1	2	3	4	5
Strongly Disagree	Disagree	Neutral	Agree	Strongly Agree

3. My wellness training has helped me to support clients at the writing center:

1	2	3	4	5
Strongly Disagree	Disagree	Neutral	Agree	Strongly Agree

4. The wellness training prompted me to develop new methods of helping others at the writing center:

1	2	3	4	5
Strongly Disagree	Disagree	Neutral	Agree	Strongly Agree

5. Wellness training changed the ways in which I handle stressful situations beyond the university setting:

1	2	3	4	5
Strongly Disagree	Disagree	Neutral	Agree	Strongly Agree

6. Wellness training has changed the ways in which I would respond to university-wide emergencies:

1	2	3	4	5
Strongly Disagree	Disagree	Neutral	Agree	Strongly Agree

7. How many times did you utilize your wellness training last semester (F16)? (please give your response in a number)

    ____ times

8. How many times did you utilize your wellness training Spring 2017 semester? (please give your response in a number)

    ____ times

9. I refer clients to wellness resources on campus:

1	2	3	4	5
rarely	sometimes	often	mostly	always

VI. Reflections on Your Current Job:

1. Writing center work gives me a sense of purpose:

1	2	3	4	5
Strongly Disagree	Disagree	Neutral	Agree	Strongly Agree

2. The Writing Center provides me with a community:

1	2	3	4	5
Strongly Disagree	Disagree	Neutral	Agree	Strongly Agree

3. My job at the writing center produces stress in my life:

1	2	3	4	5
Strongly Disagree	Disagree	Neutral	Agree	Strongly Agree

4. I am comfortable communicating with colleagues at the Writing Center:

1	2	3	4	5
Strongly Disagree	Disagree	Neutral	Agree	Strongly Agree

5. I am comfortable communicating with clients at the Writing Center:

1	2	3	4	5
Strongly Disagree	Disagree	Neutral	Agree	Strongly Agree

6. The Writing Center cares about my well-being:

1	2	3	4	5
Strongly Disagree	Disagree	Neutral	Agree	Strongly Agree

7. The Writing Center provides a positive work environment for me:

1	2	3	4	5
Strongly Disagree	Disagree	Neutral	Agree	Strongly Agree

8. I am confident handling unanticipated stressful events in the Writing Center:

1	2	3	4	5
Strongly Disagree	Disagree	Neutral	Agree	Strongly Agree

9. A culture of wellness matters to our work at the Writing Center:

1	2	3	4	5
Strongly Disagree	Disagree	Neutral	Agree	Strongly Agree

VII. Open-Ended Responses:

1. What strategies have you developed in identifying wellness needs in others? Please elaborate or provide an example.

2. Can you share an episode or event, within or outside of the Writing Center that allowed you to use any wellness training skills developed from Writing Center training?

3. What recommendations would you give for future wellness training opportunities?

Thank you for taking the time and effort to respond to this survey. We will keep you informed about the results and will continue to support wellness initiatives in future trainings.

APPENDIX C

SAMPLE OF WEEKLY MINDFULNESS EXERCISES

- **Week 1**, "Breathing Lines" exercise
- **Week 2**, Loving kindness exercise: How do you show empathy towards clients?
- **Week 3**, Mindful listening exercise: A few minutes of an Autonomous Sensory Meridian
- **Week 4**, Guided meditation activity
- **Week 5**, Guided body scan activity
- **Week 6**, Tutor intentionality discussion
- **Week 7**, Reflective writing: What do you feel gratitude about in your life?
- **Week 8**, Guided visualization activity
- **Week 9**, Mindful activity: Take 3–5 minutes to do deep breathing and/or walking
- **Week 10**, Reflective writing: Write down all that has stressed you out for the day (if anything)

https://doi.org/10.7330/9781646423606.c011

APPENDIX D

SAMPLE EMERGENCY PLAN

This emergency plan template is a general document that has been composited from a number of different sources, such as FEMA, Ohio State, Nova Scotia Department of Education, etc. A list of resources is available in references for developing an emergency plan; however, it is critical to check with your institution to see what emergency plans are already in place. It is likely that your school has a school-wide emergency plan; however, you may want to develop a departmental/unit-wide emergency plan that is specific to your unit and any satellite location(s) on campus. Because this is only a template, please ensure you share it widely with community stakeholders and emergency response teams/security professionals on campus. This should be a widely shared and revised document and it should be in a place that is accessible and public. Please also note that the nature of emergency planning is one that is recursive, ongoing, and imperfect. It is critical to acknowledge that there is no perfect emergency plan and to regularly return to these plans and update them as new events occur, new protocols and procedures are developed, and old ones are updated.

Title Page:
Sample Writing Center Emergency Plan

Include picture of main location(s)/building(s)

Name of building
Building address
Units/departments housed within the building

Next Page:
Table of Contents identifying key pertinent information in emergency
plan.

Some topics to include:

I.   Introduction to Emergency Plan/Planning
   - Signatory page indicating all departmental employees have reviewed and approved the emergency plan
   - Define an emergency

https://doi.org/10.7330/9781646423606.c012

- Explain purpose of emergency plan and scope of document
- Information about the department—number of staff, details about size and scope of department, key contact information, etc.
- Include hazard analysis summary for department/institution
- Include key pertinent information about specific site including way-finding details such as photos, signage, landmarks, etc. Information should include: location(s) on campus, proximity to other departments, resources around the site(s), and location of the following: exits, elevator, basement, fire extinguishers, first aid kit, staff contact information, safety documentation, evacuation plans, etc.
- Develop note on emergency planning and unanticipated events

II. Planning Before an Emergency

- Include emergency contact list of all personnel in department, including names, positions, emails, and phone numbers
- Include a designated main contact/person in charge, in event of an emergency
- Include departmental communication plan in the event of an emergency (i.e., how the department will communicate with employees during an emergency)
- Define key emergency planning terms (e.g., "run, hide, fight," "shelter-in-place vs. lockdown")
- Explain College-Wide Emergency Response Management System (if your school does not have an emergency response management system, immediately advocate for your institution to set one up):

  » How it works
  » How to access it
  » How to register for it/ensure you are registered

- Articulate training expectations for personnel and link to any on-line trainings (active shooter training, Title IX training, COVID-19 safety training, laboratory safety training, etc.)
- Include articulated policy for when to call campus security/police that accounts for the safety of people of color in the department

III. Employee Expectations and Responsibilities During an Emergency

- Include responsibilities for personnel in the event of an emergency
- Include policies for when to evacuate
- Include key evacuation routes, visually and textually articulated
- Identify main meet-up points in the event of evacuation, visually and textually articulated
- Articulate protocol for evacuation of persons with disabilities

IV. Evacuation Procedures

- Evacuation procedures

  » When to evacuate
  » When not to evacuate
  » What to do when evacuating

» Meeting points during an evacuation
» Planning for vacating campus in cases where emergency prohibits meeting points

Returning, Post-Evacuation

- Evacuation procedures for people with disabilities

V. Responding during Specific Emergencies (Identify Threats in Order of Likelihood):

- Distressed/disturbed individual
- Gas leak
- Fire
- Inclement weather incident (tornado, blizzard, flood, etc.)
- Active aggressor situation
- Pandemic
- Cyber attack
- Other

VI. Post-Emergency: Wellbeing and Recovery

- Resources for coping in an ongoing crisis
- Resources for coping after crisis resolution
- Debrief procedures after emergency is resolved
- Workplace policies for addressing ongoing personnel trauma
- Workplace policies for addressing ongoing chronic issues related to emergency

VII. Emergency Planning and Crisis Response Resources

- History of FEMA: https://www.fema.gov/about-agency
- Other history of FEMA: https://www.wired.com/story/the-secret -history-of-fema
- FEMA Training Guide for University Leaders: https://training.fema .gov/hiedu/aemrc/eplanning/g367.aspx
- FEMA webinars: https://training.fema.gov/hiedu/femawebinar .aspx
- FEMA training resources: https://training.fema.gov/hiedu/high links2.aspx
- FEMA emergency planning course: https://training.fema.gov/is /courseoverview.aspx?code=IS-288.a
- FEMA white paper on storytelling in emergency training education: https://training.fema.gov/hiedu/docs/latest/2020_storytelling_in _em_report.pdf

APPENDIX E

SAMPLE EMERGENCY DISCUSSION SCENARIOS

Scenario 1

You are on your way to campus when you receive an alert that there is an active shooter on campus. What do you do?

Scenario 2

You are already on campus for a mentorship group meeting when a security officer comes in and says that you are under lockdown. What do you do?

Scenario 3

You are working with a client in Smith Lab when a building coordinator comes in and tells you that there is a gas leak and that you need to evacuate the building. What do you do?

Scenario 4

You are consulting in Thompson when the tornado sirens begin to sound. What do you do?

Scenario 5

You are working with a client that is behaving erratically. They mention the pressure they feel to succeed, their poor relationship with a professor, and their personal habits—sleeping little, eating little, studying too much, etc. At one point, the client says that they would be better off dead. What do you do?

Scenario 6

You are working with a client that is physically imposing and aggressive—they are using their body in ways that make you uncomfortable, such as leaning in too close, making inappropriate comments, and, perhaps, yelling. What do you do?

Scenario 7

A person keeps coming into the writing center space to talk to consultants but they do not have an appointment and refuse to give their name. What do you do?

Scenario 8

A writer comes in and shares a personal statement that details being sexually assaulted at a party. What do you do?

https://doi.org/10.7330/9781646423606.c013

REFERENCES

"A Periodic Table of Visualization Methods." (n.d.). Retrieved September 1, 2017, from https://www.visual-literacy.org/periodic_table/periodic_table.html

Abraham, J. M. (2019). Employer wellness programs—a work in progress. *Jama, 321*(15), 1462–1463.

Adetiba, L., & Almendrala, A. (2016, July 8). *Watching videos of police brutality can traumatize you, especially if you're black.* HuffPost. https://www.huffpost.com/entry/watching-police -brutality-videos_n_577ee9b3e4b0344d514eaa5d

Afropunk. (2018, December 7). *Radical self-care: Angela Davis.* Afropunk. https://afropunk .com/2018/12/radical-self-care-angela-davis/

Alund, N. (2020, January 27). Nashville homicide victim Shawnton Clay: A 'champion of black women's health.' *Tennessean.* https://www.tennessean.com/story/news/crime/20 20/01/27/nashville-homicide-victim-shawnton-clay/4587173002/

American Psychological Association. (2020). *Sample tables.* APA Style. https://apastyle.apa .org/style-grammar-guidelines/tables-figures/sample-tables

Anderson, G. (2020, September 11). *Mental health needs rise with pandemic.* Inside Higher Ed. https://www.insidehighered.com/news/2020/09/11/students-great-need-mental -health-support-during-pandemic

Arismunandar, A., & Emmiyati, N. (2016). Work stress and psychological consequences in the workplace: Study on elementary school teachers. *Jurnal Ilmu Pendidikan, 10*(3).

Atkinson, P. B. (2011). Exploring correlations between writing apprehension, academic rational beliefs, and stress and coping behaviors in college students. *Proceedings of the New York State Communication Association, 2010*(1), 1–24.

Babcock, R. D., & Thonus, T. (2012). *Researching the writing center: Towards an evidence-based practice.* Peter Lang.

Bandura, A. (2006). Guide for creating self-efficacy scales. In F. Pajares & T. Urdan (Eds.), *Self-efficacy beliefs of adolescents* (pp. 307–337). Information Age Publishing.

Barbezat, D. P., & Bush, M. (2013). *Contemplative practices in higher education: Powerful methods to transform teaching and learning.* John Wiley & Sons.

Bartlett, L., Martin, A., Neil, A. L., Memish, K., Otahal, P., Kilpatrick, M., & Sanderson, K. (2019). A systematic review and meta-analysis of workplace mindfulness training randomized controlled trials. *Journal of Occupational Health Psychology, 24*(1), 108.

Beck, A. J., Hirth, R. A., Jenkins, K. R., Sleeman, K. K., & Zhang, W. (2016). Factors associated with participation in a university worksite wellness program. *American Journal of Preventive Medicine, 51*(1), e1–e11.

Beck, J. (2018, November 26). The concept creep of 'emotional labor.' *The Atlantic.* https:// www.theatlantic.com/family/archive/2018/11/arlie-hochschild-housework-isnt-emo tional-labor/576637/

Becker, D., & Marecek, J. (2008). Positive psychology: History in the remaking? *Theory & Psychology, 18*(5), 591–604.

Berger, M., & Sarnyai, Z. (2015). "More than skin deep": Stress neurobiology and mental health consequences of racial discrimination. *Stress, 18*(1), 1–10.

Black, L. L., Johnson, R., & VanHoose, L. (2015). The relationship between perceived racism/discrimination and health among black American women: A review of the literature from 2003 to 2013. *Journal of Racial and Ethnic Health Disparities, 2*(1), 11–20.

https://doi.org/10.7330/9781646423606.c014

Body Politic. (2020). *About us.* Body Politic. Retrieved June 1, 2020, from https://www.weare bodypolitic.com/about-body-politic

Boquet, E. H. (1999). "Our little secret": A history of writing centers, pre-to post-open admissions. *College Composition and Communication, 50*(3), 463–482.

brown, a. m. (2019). *Pleasure activism: The politics of feeling good.* AK Press.

Bruffee, K. A. (1984). Collaborative learning and the "conversation of mankind." *College English, 46*(7), 635–652.

Bruxvoort, D. (2012). Disaster preparedness for colleges and universities. *Texas Library Journal, 88*(3), 100.

Busso, D. S., McLaughlin, K. A., & Sheridan, M. A. (2014). Media exposure and sympathetic nervous system reactivity predict PTSD symptoms after the Boston marathon bombings. *Depression and Anxiety, 31*(7), 551–558.

Call, C., Gerdes, R., & Robinson, K. (2009, March 27). *Health and wellness research study: Corporate and worksite wellness programs: A research review focused on individuals with disabilities* (Government Contract No. DOLU089428186). Social Dynamics, LLC. http://www.dol .gov/odep/research/CorporateWellnessResearchLiteratureReview.pdf

Canning, J. (2014). *Statistics for the humanities.* Creative Commons. http://statistics forhumanities.net/book/

Carino, P. (1995). Early writing centers: Toward a history. *The Writing Center Journal, 15*(2), 103–115.

Carter, S. (2009). The writing center paradox: Talk about legitimacy and the problem of institutional change. *College Composition and Communication, 61*(1), W133.

Carter-Tod, S. (2020) Administrating while black: Negotiating the emotional labor of an African American WPA. In C. Wooten, J. Babb, K. Murray Costello & K. Navickas (Eds.), *The things we carry: Strategies for recognizing and negotiating emotional labor in writing program administration* (pp. 309–310). Utah State University Press.

Cassar, V., Bezzina, F., Fabri, S., & Buttigieg, S. C. (2020). Work stress in the 21st century: A bibliometric scan of the first 2 decades of research in this millennium. *Society of Psychologists in Management. The Psychologist-Manager Journal, 23*(2), 47–75.

Caswell, N., McKinney, J. G., & Jackson, R. (2016). *The working lives of new writing center directors.* Utah State University Press.

Chandler, S. (2007). Fear, teaching composition, and students' discursive choices: Rethinking connections between emotions and college student writing. *Composition Studies, 35*(2), 53–70.

Clinnin, K. (2020). And so I respond: The emotional labor of writing program administrators in crisis response. In C. Wooten, J. Babb, K. Murray Costello & K. Navickas (Eds.), *The things we carry: Strategies for recognizing and negotiating emotional labor in writing program administration* (pp. 129–144). Utah State University Press.

Cole, H. A., Prassel, H. B., & Carlson, C. R. (2018). A meta-analysis of computer-delivered drinking interventions for college students: A comprehensive review of studies from 2010 to 2016. *Journal of Studies on Alcohol and Drugs, 79*(5), 686–696.

Collins, P. H. (1989). The social construction of black feminist thought. *Signs: Journal of women in culture and society, 14*(4), 745–773.

Concannon, K., Morris, J., Chavannes, N., & Diaz, V. (2020). Cultivating emotional wellness and self-care through mindful mentorship in the writing center. *WLN: A Journal of Writing Center Scholarship, 44*(5–6), 10–18.

Condon, F. (2007). Beyond the known: Writing centers and the work of anti-racism. *The Writing Center Journal, 27*(2), 19–38.

Conference on College Composition & Communication (CCCC). (2015, November). *Guidelines for the ethical conduct of research in composition studies.* Conference on College Composition & Communication. https://cccc.ncte.org/cccc/resources/positions/ethical conduct

Conference on College Composition & Communication (CCCC), & CWPA. (2020, June). *Joint statement in response to the COVID-19 pandemic.* Conference on College Composition & Communication. https://cccc.ncte.org/cccc/cccc-and-cwpa-joint-statement-in-response-to-the-covid-19-pandemic

Consilio, J., & Kennedy, S. M. (2019). Using mindfulness as a heuristic for writing evaluation: Transforming pedagogy and quality of experience. *Across the Disciplines, 16*(1), 28–49.

Costello, K. M. (2021). Naming and negotiating the emotional labors of writing center tutoring. In G. Giaimo (Ed.), *Wellness and care in writing center work.* WLN.

Cramer, R. J., Ireland, J. L., Hartley, V., Long, M. M., Ireland, C. A., & Wilkins, T. (2020). Coping, mental health, and subjective well-being among mental health staff working in secure forensic psychiatric settings: Results from a workplace health assessment. *Psychological services, 17*(2), 160–169.

Dailey, S. L., Burke, T. J., & Carberry, E. G. (2018). For better or for work: Dual discourses in a workplace wellness program. *Management Communication Quarterly, 32*(4), 612–626.

Daly, J., & Miller, M. (1975). The empirical development of an instrument to measure writing apprehension. *Research in the Teaching of English, 9*(3), 242–249.

Degner, H., Wojciehowski, K., & Giroux, C. (2015). Opening closed doors: A rationale for creating a safe space for tutors struggling with mental health concerns or illnesses. *Praxis: A Writing Center Journal.*

Denny, H., Nordlof, J., & Salem, L. (2018). "Tell me exactly what it was that I was doing that was so bad": Understanding the needs and expectations of working-class students in writing centers. *The Writing Center Journal, 37*(1), 67–100.

DeRango-Adem, A. (2017, November 30). *Self-care is a radical act, but not in the way we're practising it right now.* FLARE. https://www.flare.com/living/self-care-is-a-radical-act/

Diab, R., Godbee, B., Ferrel, T., & Simpkins, N. (2012). A multi-dimensional pedagogy for racial justice in writing centers. *Praxis: A Writing Center Journal.*

Driscoll, D. L., & Wells, J. (2012). Beyond knowledge and skills: Writing transfer and the role of student dispositions. *Composition Forum, 26.*

Ehrenreich, B., & English, D. (2005). *For her own good: Two centuries of the experts' advice to women.* Anchor.

Emmelhainz, N. (2020). Tutoring begins with breath: Guided meditation and its effects on writing consultant training. *WLN: A Journal of Writing Center Scholarship, 44*(5–6), 2–10.

Estrin, J. (2020, July 15). Their workers kept being stopped by the police, so they decided to help. *The New York Times.* https://www.nytimes.com/2020/07/15/nyregion/grand-champs-brooklyn-black-lives-matter.html?action=click&module=Top%20Stories&pgtype=Homepage

European Agency for Safety and Health at Work (2020). *Psychosocial risks and stress at work.* European Agency for Safety and Health at Work. https://osha.europa.eu/en/themes/psychosocial-risks-and-stress

Evans, L., & Moore, W. L. (2015). Impossible burdens: White institutions, emotional labor, and micro-resistance. *Social Problems, 62*(3), 439–454.

Faison, W. (2018). Black bodies, black language: Exploring the use of black language as a tool of survival in the writing center. *The Peer Review, 2*(1).

Faison, W. (2019). Writing as a practice of freedom: HBCU writing centers as sites of Liberatory practice. *Praxis: A Writing Center Journal.*

Faison, W., & Treviño, A. (2017). Race, retention, language, and literacy: The hidden curriculum of the writing center. *The Peer Review, 1*(2).

Featherstone, J., Barrett, R., & Chandler, M. (2019). The mindful tutor. In K. G. Johnson & T. Roggenbuck (Eds.), *WLN digital edited collection.* wlnjournal.org/digitaleditedcollection1/

Federal Emergency Management Institute (FEMA). (2015). *The role of voluntary organizations in emergency management.* FEMA. https://training.fema.gov/is/courseoverview.aspx?co

de=is-288.a#:~:text=Today%2C%20they%20serve%20a%20critical,and%20long %2Dterm%20recovery%20services

Fifolt, M., Burrowes, J., McPherson, T., & McCormick, L. C. (2016). Strengthening emergency preparedness in higher education through hazard vulnerability analysis. *College and University, 91*(4), 61.

Fisher, D. M., Kerr, A. J., & Cunningham, S. (2019). Examining the moderating effect of mindfulness on the relationship between job stressors and strain outcomes. *International Journal of Stress Management, 26*(1), 78.

Fitzpatrick, A. J. (2021). Undergraduate unionization: A new frontier of student organizing in a post-Columbia world. *Iowa Law Review, 106*(3), 1393.

Franzidis, A. F., & Zinder, S. M. (2019). Examining student wellness for the development of campus-based wellness programs. *Building Healthy Academic Communities Journal, 3*(1), 56–66.

Gamache, P. (2003). Zen and the art of the writing tutorial. *The Writing Lab Newsletter, 28*(2), 1–4.

García, R. (2017). Unmaking gringo-centers. *The Writing Center Journal, 29*–60.

Garza, A. (2020). *The purpose of power: How we come together when we fall apart.* One World.

Geller, A. E., & Denny, H. (2013). Of ladybugs, low status, and loving the job: Writing center professionals navigating their careers. *The Writing Center Journal, 33*(1), 96–129.

Ghannam, J., Afana, A., Ho, E. Y., Al-Khal, A., & Bylund, C. L. (2020). The impact of a stress management intervention on medical residents' stress and burnout. *International Journal of Stress Management, 27*(1), 65–73.

Giaimo, G. (2017). Focusing on the blind spots: RAD-based assessment of students' perceptions of a community college writing center. *Praxis: A Writing Center Journal.*

Giaimo, G. (2019). Where theory and praxis collide: Supporting student-led writing center research at two-year colleges. *Teaching English in the Two-Year College, 46*(4), 297–316.

Giaimo, G. (2020). Laboring in a time of crisis: The entanglement of wellness and work in writing centers. *Praxis: A Writing Center Journal, 17*(3), 1–12.

Giaimo, G. (2021). A matter of method: Wellness and care research in writing center studies by Genie Nicole Giaimo. In G. N. Giaimo (Ed.), *Wellness and care in writing center work.* WLN: A Journal of Writing Center Scholarship, Digital Edited Collections.

Giaimo, G. N., Cheatle, J. J., Hastings, C. K., & Modley, C. (2018). It's all in the notes: What session notes can tell us about the work of writing centers. *Journal of Writing Analytics, 2*, 225–256.

Giaimo, G. & Hashlamon, Y. (Eds.). (2020). Wellness and care special issue. *WLN: A Journal of Writing Center Scholarship, 44*(5–6).

Gillespie, P., & Lerner, N. (2008). *The Longman guide to peer tutoring.* Longman Publishing Group.

GirlTrek (2020). *Our mission.* GirlTrek. https://www.girltrek.org/

Global Wellness Institute. (2020). *What is the wellness economy?* Global Wellness Institute. https://globalwellnessinstitute.org/what-is-wellness/what-is-the-wellness-economy/

Gorski, P. C. (2015). Relieving burnout and the "martyr syndrome" among social justice education activists: The implications and effects of mindfulness. *The Urban Review, 47*(4), 696–716.

Gorski, P. C. (2019). Fighting racism, battling burnout: Causes of activist burnout in US racial justice activists. *Ethnic and Racial Studies, 42*(5), 667–687.

Graf, E. M., Sator, M., & Spranz-Fogasy, T. (Eds.). (2014). *Discourses of helping professions* (Vol. 252). John Benjamins Publishing Company.

Green, N. A. (2018). Moving beyond alright: And the emotional toll of this, my life matters too, in the writing center work. *The Writing Center Journal, 37*(1), 15–34.

Gunther, J. (2018, August 1). Worshipping the false idols of wellness. *The New York Times.* https://www.nytimes.com/2018/08/01/style/wellness-industrial-complex.html

Gutteling, J. M. (2000). Current views on risk communication and their implications for crisis and reputation management. *Document Design, 2*(3), 236–246.

Hall, R. M. (2017). *Around the texts of writing center work: An inquiry-based approach to tutor education.* Utah State University Press.

Haltiwanger Morrison, T. M., & Nanton, T. O. (2019). Dear writing centers: Black women speaking silence into language and action. *The Peer Review, 3*(1).

Harrell, J. P., Hall, S., & Taliaferro, J. (2003). Physiological responses to racism and discrimination: An assessment of the evidence. *American Journal of Public Health, 93*(2), 243–248.

Harris, A. (2017, April 5). *A history of self-care: From its radical roots to its yuppie-driven middle age to its election-inspired resurgence.* Slate. http://www.slate.com/articles/arts/cul turebox/2017/04/the_history_of_self_care.html

Harris, M. (1995). Talking in the middle: Why writers need writing tutors. *College English, 57*(1), 27–42.

Harrison, M. E. (2012). The power of "no": Buddhist mindfulness and the teaching of composition. *Writing on the Edge, 22*(2), 36–46.

Healy, D. (1991). Tutorial role conflict in the writing center. *The Writing Center Journal, 11*(2), 41–50.

Healy, D. (1995). Writing center directors: An emerging portrait of the profession. *Writing Program Administration, 18*(3), 26–43.

Heckelman, R. (1998). The writing center as managerial site. *Writing Lab Newsletter, 23*(1), 1–4.

Henkey, T. (2017). *Urban emergency management: Planning and response for the 21st century.* Butterworth-Heinemann.

Hermann, J. (2017). Brave/r spaces vs. safe spaces for LGBTQ+ in the writing center: Theory and practice at the University of Kansas. *The Peer Review, 1*(2).

Hill, E. M., LaLonde, C. M., & Reese, L. A. (2020). Compassion fatigue in animal care workers. *Traumatology, 26*(1), 96–108.

Hings, R. F., Wagstaff, C. R., Anderson, V., Gilmore, S., & Thelwell, R. C. (2020). Better preparing sports psychologists for the demands of applied practice: The emotional labor training gap. *Journal of Applied Sport Psychology, 32*(4), 335–356.

Hochschild, A. R. (1979). Emotion work, feeling rules, and social structure. *American Journal of Sociology, 85*(3), 551–575.

Hochschild, A. R. (2012). *The managed heart: Commercialization of human feeling.* University of California Press.

hooks, b. (2000). *All about love: New visions.* Harper Perennial.

Hughes, B., Gillespie, P., & Kail, H. (2010). What they take with them: Findings from the peer writing tutor alumni research project. *The Writing Center Journal, 30*(2), 12–46.

Huxter, M. (2015). Mindfulness and the Buddha's noble eightfold path. In *Buddhist foundations of mindfulness* (pp. 29–53). Springer.

Ianetta, M., & Fitzgerald, L. (2016). *The Oxford guide for writing tutors: Practice and research.* Oxford University Press.

Inoue, A. B. (2015). *Antiracist writing assessment ecologies: Teaching and assessing writing for a socially just future.* Parlor Press LLC.

James, E. P., & Zoller, H. M. (2018). Resistance training: (Re)shaping extreme forms of workplace health promotion. *Management Communication Quarterly, 32*(1), 60–89.

Jarman, L., Martin, A., Venn, A., Otahal, P., & Sanderson, K. (2015). Does workplace health promotion contribute to job stress reduction? Three-year findings from Partnering Healthy@ Work. *BMC Public Health, 15*(1), 1293.

Jenkins, K. R., Fakhoury, N., Richardson, C. R., Segar, M., Krupka, E., & Kullgren, J. (2019). Characterizing employees' preferences for incentives for healthy behaviors: Examples to improve interest in wellness programs. *Health Promotion Practice, 20*(6), 880–889.

Jerolleman, A. (2020). *Exploring the current and future uses of storytelling in emergency management education*. FEMA.

Johnson, S. (2018). Mindful tutors, embodied writers: Positioning mindfulness meditation as a writing strategy to optimize cognitive load and potentialize writing center tutors' supportive roles. *Praxis: A Writing Center Journal.*

Jordan, J. (1995). *Civil wars*. Simon and Schuster.

Kabat-Zinn, J. (2003). Mindfulness-based stress reduction (MBSR). *Constructivism in the Human Sciences, 8*(2), 73.

Kabat-Zinn, J. (2011). Some reflections on the origins of MBSR, skillful means, and the trouble with maps. *Contemporary Buddhism, 12*(1), 281–306.

Kabat-Zinn, J., Lipworth, L., Burney, R., & Sellers, W. (1987). Four-year follow-up of a meditation-based program for the self-regulation of chronic pain: Treatment outcomes and compliance. *The Clinical Journal of Pain, 3*(1), 60,

Kapucu, N., & Khosa, S. (2013). Disaster resiliency and culture of preparedness for university and college campuses. *Administration & Society, 45*(1), 3–37.

Kim, W. O. (2012). Institutional review board (IRB) and ethical issues in clinical research. *Korean Journal of Anesthesiology, 62*(1), 3.

Kinane, K. (2019). The place of practice in contemplative pedagogy and writing. *Across the Disciplines, 16*(1), 6–15.

Kinkead, J. (2015). *Researching writing: An introduction to research methods*. Utah State University Press.

Kisner, J. (2017, March 14). The politics of conspicuous displays of self-care. *The New Yorker*. https://www.newyorker.com/culture/culture-desk/the-politics-of-selfcare

Klein, N. (2007). *The shock doctrine: The rise of disaster capitalism*. Macmillan.

Klingbeil, D. A., & Renshaw, T. L. (2018). Mindfulness-based interventions for teachers: A meta-analysis of the emerging evidence base. *School Psychology Quarterly, 33*(4), 501.

Kroll, K. (2008). On paying attention: Flagpoles, mindfulness, and teaching writing. *Teaching English in the Two-Year College, 36*(1), 69.

Kvatum, L. (2020, September 8). Why human brains are bad at assessing the risks of pandemics. *The Washington Post*. https://www.washingtonpost.com/lifestyle/magazine/why-human-brains-are-bad-at-assessing-the-risks-of-pandemics/2020/09/03/7395321c-dd9d-11ea-b205-ff838e15a9a6_story.html

Lavelle, E. (2010). Writing through college: Self-efficacy and instruction. In R. Beard, D. Myhill, J. Riley & M. Nystrand (Eds.), *The sage handbook of writing development* (pp. 415–422). Sage.

Lawson, D. (2015). Metaphors and ambivalence: Affective dimensions in writing center studies. *WLN: A Journal of Writing Center Scholarship, 40*(3–4), 20–28.

Lee, Y. H. (2019). Emotional labor, teacher burnout, and turnover intention in high-school physical education teaching. *European Physical Education Review, 25*(1), 236–253.

Lindqvist, H., Weurlander, M., Wernerson, A., & Thornberg, R. (2019). Boundaries as a coping strategy: Emotional labour and relationship maintenance in distressing teacher education situations. *European Journal of Teacher Education, 42*(5), 634–649.

Liu, H., Mattke, S., Harris, K. M., Weinberger, S., Serxner, S., Caloyeras, J. P., & Exum, E. (2013). Do workplace wellness programs reduce medical costs? Evidence from a Fortune 500 company. *Inquiry: The Journal of Health Care Organization, Provision, and Financing, 50*(2), 150–158.

Lloyd, L. K., Crixell, S. H., Bezner, J. R., Forester, K., & Swearingen, C. (2017). Genesis of an employee wellness program at a large university. *Health Promotion Practice, 18*(6), 879–894.

Lorde, A. (2017). *A burst of light: And other essays*. Courier Dover Publications.

Lowenstein, F. (2020, March 23). I'm 26. Coronavirus sent me to the hospital. *The New York Times*. https://www.nytimes.com/2020/03/23/opinion/coronavirus-young-people.html

Mack, E., & Hupp, K. (2017). Mindfulness in the writing Ccnter: A total encounter. *Praxis: A Writing Center Journal.*

Mackiewicz, J., & Babcock, R. (Eds.). (2019). *Theories and methods of writing center studies: A practical guide.* Routledge.

Maex, E. (2011). The Buddhist roots of mindfulness training: A practitioners view. *Contemporary Buddhism, 12*(1), 165–175.

Mahdawi, A. (2017, January 12). Generation treat yo' self: The problem with 'self-care.' *The Guardian.* https://www.theguardian.com/lifeandstyle/2017/jan/12/self-care-problems-solange-knowles

Maslach, C., Schaufeli, W. B., & Leiter, M. P. (2001). Job burnout. *Annual Review of Psychology, 52*(1), 397–422.

Mathieu, P. (2016). Being there: Mindfulness as ethical classroom practice. *The Journal of the Assembly for Expanded Perspectives on Learning, 21*(1), 5.

McCabe, A. (2020, June 16). *GirlTrek uses black women's history to encourage walking as a healing tradition.* National Public Radio. https://www.npr.org/2020/06/16/877100939/girltrek-uses-black-womens-history-to-encourage-walking-as-a-healing-tradition.

McKinney, J. G. (2005). Leaving home sweet home: Towards critical readings of writing center spaces. *The Writing Center Journal, 25*(2), 6–20.

McKinney, J. G. (2015). *Strategies for writing center research.* Parlor Press.

McNamarah, C. T. (2019). White caller crime: Racialized police communication and existing while black. *Michigan Journal of Race and Law, 24*(2), 335.

Miller, W. R., & Rollnick, S. (2004). Talking oneself into change: Motivational interviewing, stages of change, and therapeutic process. *Journal of Cognitive Psychotherapy, 18*(4), 299–308.

Mirk, S. (2016, February 18). Audre Lorde thought of self-Ccre as an "act of political warfare." *Bitch Media.* https://www.bitchmedia.org/article/audre-lorde-thought-self-care-act-political-warfare

Monty, R. (2019). Undergirding writing centers' responses to the neoliberal academy. *Praxis: A Writing Center Journal.*

Moore, C. (2018). Mentoring WPAs for the long term: The promise of mindfulness. *WPA: Writing Program Administration-Journal of the Council of Writing Program Administrators, 42*(1).

Morrow, D. S. (1991). Tutoring writing: Healing or what? *College Composition and Communication, 42*(2), 218–229.

Mueller, D. N. (2017). *Network sense: Methods for visualizing a discipline.* WAC Clearinghouse.

Murphy, C. (1989). Freud in the writing center: The psychoanalytics of tutoring well. *The Writing Center Journal, 10*(1), 13–18.

Murray, D. (2003, June). Zen tutoring: Unlocking the mind. *The Writing Lab Newsletter, 27*(10), 12–14. https://wlnjournal.org/archives/v27/27.10.pdf

Nash, J. C. (2013). Practicing love: Black feminism, love-politics, and post-intersectionality. *Meridians, 11*(2), 1–24.

National Institute for Occupation Safety and Health (NIOSH). (2020). *Stress at work.* Center for Disease Control and Prevention. https://www.cdc.gov/niosh/docs/99-101/default.html#What%20Is%20Job%20Stress?

Nelson, J. (2015). *More than medicine: A history of the feminist women's health movement.* NYU Press.

Nelson, S., Burns, M., McEwen, B., & Borsook, D. (2020). Stressful experiences in youth: "Set-up" for diminished resilience to chronic pain. *Brain, Behavior, & Immunity-Health, 5,* 100095.

New York Times. (n.d.). *Bringing wellness to your life: Learn how to improve yourself and your relationships.* New York Times Style Section. Retrieved December 10, 2019, from https://www.nytimes.com/spotlight/bringing-wellness-to-your-life

Nicklay, J. (2012). Got guilt? Consultant guilt in the writing center community. *The Writing Center Journal, 32*(1), 14–27.

Nyman, J. A., Barleen, N. A., & Abraham, J. M. (2010). The effectiveness of health promotion at the University of Minnesota: Expenditures, absenteeism, and participation in specific programs. *Journal of Occupational and Environmental Medicine, 52*(3), 269–280.

Olssen, M., & Peters, M. A. (2005). Neoliberalism, higher education and the knowledge economy: From the free market to knowledge capitalism. *Journal of Education Policy, 20*(3), 313–345.

Palenchar, M. J. (2009). Historical trends of risk and crisis communication. *Handbook of Risk and Crisis Communication,* 31–52.

Parsons, K. (2020). Tutors' column: Just say 'no': Setting emotional boundaries in the writing center is a practice in self-care. *WLN: A Journal of Writing Center Scholarship, 44*(5–6), 26–30.

Perdue, S. W., Driscoll, D. L., & Petrykowski, A. (2017). Centering institutional status and scholarly identity: An analysis of writing center administration position advertisements, 2004–2014. *The Writing Center Journal, 36*(2), 265–293.

Perry, A. (2016). Training for triggers: Helping writing center consultants navigate emotional sessions. *Composition Forum,* (34).

Piazza, C., & Siebert, C. (2008). Development and validation of a writing dispositions scale for elementary and middle school students. *The Journal of Educational Research, 101,* 275–285.

Positive Psychology Center. (n.d.). *Our mission.* University of Pennsylvania. Retrieved October 10, 2018, from https://ppc.sas.upenn.edu/our-mission

Prochaska, J. O., & DiClemente, C. C. (1982). Transtheoretical therapy: Toward a more integrative model of change. *Psychotherapy: Theory, Research & Practice, 19*(3), 276.

Prochaska, J. O., DiClemente, C. C., & Norcross, J. C. (1993). In search of how people change: Applications to addictive behaviors. *Addictions Nursing Network, 5*(1), 2–16.

Ratnayake, S. (2019, July 25). The problem of mindfulness. *Aeon.* Retrieved from https://aeon.co/essays/mindfulness-is-loaded-with-troubling-metaphysical-assumptions?utm_source=pocket-newtab

Regehr, C., Nelson, S., & Hildyard, A. (2017). Academic continuity planning in higher education. *Journal of Business Continuity & Emergency Planning, 11*(1), 73–84.

Roeser, R. W., Schonert-Reichl, K. A., Jha, A., Cullen, M., Wallace, L., Wilensky, R., & Harrison, J. (2013). Mindfulness training and reductions in teacher stress and burnout: Results from two randomized, waitlist-control field trials. *Journal of Educational Psychology, 105*(3), 787.

Rogers, Kenny. (1978). The gambler [Song]. On *The Gambler.* United Artists Records.

Rowell, C. (2015). *Let's talk emotions: Re-envisioning the writing center through consultant emotional labor.* East Carolina University.

Sanchez-Reilly, S., Morrison, L. J., Carey, E., Bernacki, R., O'Neill, L., Kapo, J., & Thomas, J. D. (2013). Caring for oneself to care for others: Physicians and their self-care. *The Journal of Supportive Oncology, 11*(2), 75.

Sano-Franchini, J. (2016). "It's like writing yourself into a codependent relationship with someone who doesn't even want you!" Emotional labor, intimacy, and the academic job market in rhetoric and composition. *College Composition and Communication,* 98–124.

Sattler, D. N., Kirsch, J., Shipley, G., Cocke, P., & Stegmeier, R. (2014). Emergency preparedness on campus: Improving procedural knowledge and response readiness. *Journal of Homeland Security and Emergency Management, 11*(2), 257–268.

Satya. (2019, May 6). *Reclaiming your power thru radical self care.* Afropunk. https://afropunk.com/2019/05/reclaiming-your-power-thru-radical-self-care/

Saunders, D. B. (2010). Neoliberal ideology and public higher education in the United States. *Journal for Critical Education Policy Studies, 8*(1), 41–77.

Sauter, S. (2007, December 3). Workplace stress. *NIOSH Science Blog.* https://blogs.cdc .gov/niosh-science-blog/2007/12/03/stress/

Schlachte, C. (2020). Shelter in place: Contingency and affect in graduate teacher training courses. In C. Wooten, J. Babb, K. Murray Costello & K. Navickas (Eds.), *The things we carry: Strategies for recognizing and negotiating emotional labor in writing program administration* (pp. 145–160). Utah State University Press.

Schloss, P. J., & Cragg, K. M. (2013). The nature and role of budget processes. In P. J. Schloss & K. M. Cragg (Eds.), *Organization and administration in higher education* (pp. 119–142). Routledge.

Schmidt, K. M., & Alexander, J. E. (2012). The empirical development of an instrument to measure writerly self-efficacy in writing centers. *Journal of Writing Assessment, 5*(1), 1–10.

Schueths, A. M., Gladney, T., Crawford, D. M., Bass, K. L., & Moore, H. A. (2013). Passionate pedagogy and emotional labor: Students' responses to learning diversity from diverse instructors. *International Journal of Qualitative Studies in Education, 26*(10), 1259–1276.

Seligman, M. E., & Csikszentmihalyi, M. (2014). Positive psychology: An introduction. In *Flow and the foundations of positive psychology: The collected works of Mihaly Csikszentmihalyi* (pp. 279–298). Springer, Dordrecht.

Sherwood, S. (1995). The dark side of the helping personality: Student dependency and the potential for tutor burnout. In B. Stay, C. Murphy & E. Hobson (Eds.), *Writing center perspectives* (pp. 63–70). National Writing Centers Association Press.

Simmons, E., Miller, L. K., Prendergast, C., & McGuigan, C. (2020). Is tutoring stressful?: Measuring tutors' cortisol levels. *WLN: A Journal of Writing Center Scholarship, 44*(5–6), 18–26.

Song, Z., & Baicker, K. (2019). Effect of a workplace wellness program on employee health and economic outcomes: A randomized clinical trial. *Jama, 321*(15), 1491–1501.

Spicer, A. (2019, August 21). Self-care: How a radical feminist idea was stripped of politics for the mass market. *The Guardian.* https://www.theguardian.com/commentisfree/2019 /aug/21/self-care-radical-feminist-idea-mass-market

Spohrer, E. (2008). From goals to intentions: Yoga, zen, and our writing center work. *The Writing Lab Newsletter, 33*(2), 10–13.

Stoewen, D. L. (2017). Dimensions of wellness: Change your habits, change your life. *The Canadian Veterinary Journal, 58*(8), 861.

Strand, S. (1996, September). Book review [Review of the book *Writing center perspectives*, by B. L. Stay, C. Murphy & E. H. Hobson, Eds.]. *WLN: Journal of Writing Center Scholarship, 21*(1), 11–12.

Strickland, D. (2011). *The managerial unconscious in the history of composition studies.* SIU Press.

Sun, J., Wang, Y., Wan, Q., & Huang, Z. (2019). Mindfulness and special education teachers' burnout: The serial multiple mediation effects of self-acceptance and perceived stress. *Social Behavior and Personality: an international journal, 47*(11), 1–8.

Tarrasch, R. (2019). Mindfulness for education students: Addressing welfare as part of the professional training. *Educational Studies, 45*(3), 372–389.

Taylor, S. R. (2018). *The body is not an apology: The power of radical self-love.* Berrett-Koehler Publishers.

The Establishment. (2016, July 26). *How revolutionary self-care becomes an act of radical activism.* Afropunk. https://afropunk.com/2016/07/op-ed-how-revolutionary-self-care -becomes-an-act-of-radical-activism/

The Ohio State University. (2017). *9 dimensions of wellness.* Student Wellness Center. Retrieved March 12, 2020, from https://swc.osu.edu/about-us/9-dimensions-of-well ness/

The Ohio State University. (2017). *Wellness assessment.* Student Wellness Center. Retrieved March 12, 2020, from https://swc.osu.edu/get-involved/wellness-assessment/

The Ohio State University. (2019). *Emergency procedures.* Department of Public Safety. Retrieved March 12, 2020, from https://dps.osu.edu/emergency-procedures

The Ohio State University. (n.d.). *Guide to assist disruptive or distressed individuals.* The Office of Academic Affairs. Retrieved March 12, 2020, from https://odi.osu.edu/guide -assist-disruptive-or-distressed-individuals

Vazquez, E. M., & Levin, J. S. (2018). The tyranny of neoliberalism in the American academic profession. *American Association of University Professors* (January–February 2018). https://www.aaup.org/article/tyranny-neoliberalism-american-academic-profession# .Y1gc9XbMI2w

VIA Institute on Character. (n.d.). *About VIA survey.* Retrieved March 12, 2020, from https://www.viacharacter.org/about

Vinson, A. H., & Underman, K. (2020). Clinical empathy as emotional labor in medical work. *Social Science & Medicine,* 112904.

Washington Post Live. (2021, February 25). Be well: Wellness technology. *The Washington Post.* https://www.washingtonpost.com/washington-post-live/2021/02/25/be-well -wellness-technology/

Wenger, C. I. (2014). Feminism, mindfulness and the small university jWPA. *WPA: Writing Program Administration-Journal of the Council of Writing Program Administrators, 37*(2).

Wenger, C. I. (2015). *Yoga minds, writing bodies: Contemplative writing pedagogy.* WAC Clearinghouse.

West, E. (2019, December 14). *Socialists need to take back the term 'emotional labor'.* Jacobin. https://www.jacobinmag.com/2019/12/emotional-labor-arlie-hochschild-silvia -federici-wages-housework

Westphal, M., Bingisser, M. B., Feng, T., Wall, M., Blakley, E., Bingisser, R., & Kleim, B. (2015). Protective benefits of mindfulness in emergency room personnel. *Journal of Affective Disorders, 175,* 79–85.

Williams, M. & Delapp, R. (2016, July 14). *Tuning out: Repeated exposure to racial violence can trigger the same symptoms as PTSD. Give yourself a break.* Slate. https://slate.com/technol ogy/2016/07/when-racial-violence-happens-its-just-as-important-to-tune-out-as-it-is-to -tune-in.html

Wooten, C. A., Babb, J., Costello, K. M., & Navickas, K. (Eds.). (2020). *The things we carry: Strategies for recognizing and negotiating emotional labor in writing program administration.* Utah State University Press.

Yu, X., Wang, P., Zhai, X., Dai, H., & Yang, Q. (2015). The effect of work stress on job burnout among teachers: The mediating role of self-efficacy. *Social Indicators Research, 122*(3), 701–708.

Zaretsky, R., & Katz, Y. J. (2019). The relationship between teachers' perceptions of emotional labor and teacher burnout and teachers' educational level. *Athens Journal of Education, 6*(2), 127–144.

INDEX

Page numbers followed by *f* indicate figures. Page numbers followed by *t* indicate tables.

ABOUT THE AUTHOR

Genie Nicole Giaimo is assistant professor and director of the Writing Center at Middlebury College in Vermont. Their work has been published in *Praxis, Journal of Writing Research, The Journal of Writing Analytics, Teaching English in the Two-Year College, Research in Online Literacy Education, Kairos, Across the Disciplines, Journal of Multimodal Rhetorics*, as well as several edited collections (Utah State University Press, Parlor Press). They are also the editor of *Wellness and Care in Writing Center Work*, an open-access digital book. Giaimo is past president of Northeast Writing Center Association, past vice president of ECWCA, and past co-chair of the IWCA Summer Research Institute and Research Collaborative. Their current research utilizes quantitative and qualitative models to answer a range of questions about behaviors and practices in and around writing centers, such as tutor professional development trajectories, writing placement ethics and methods, and STEM students' writing networks and confidences. Currently based in Vermont, Genie likes open water swimming, hiking, and advocating for fair labor practices in higher education workplaces.